MCQs in Physiology

MCQs in Physiology

C.A. Browne
Senior Lecturer
Department of Physiology
Monash University
Australia

and

A. R. Luff
Associate Professor
Department of Physiology
Monash University
Australia

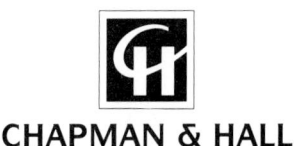

CHAPMAN & HALL
London · Weinheim · New York · Tokyo · Melbourne · Madras

Published by Chapman & Hall, 2–6 Boundary Row, London SE1 8HN, UK

Chapman & Hall, 2–6 Boundary Row, London SE1 8HN, UK

Chapman & Hall GmbH, Pappelallee 3, 69469 Weinheim, Germany

Chapman & Hall USA, 115 Fifth Avenue, New York, NY 10003, USA

Chapman & Hall Japan, ITP-Japan, Kyowa Building, 3F, 2-2-1 Hirakawacho, Chiyoda-ku, Tokyo 102, Japan

Chapman & Hall Australia, 102 Dodds Street, South Melbourne, Victoria 3205, Australia

Chapman & Hall India, R. Seshadri, 32 Second Main Road, CIT East, Madras 600 035, India

First edition 1996

© 1996 Chris Browne and Tony Luff

Typeset in 9.5/11pt Times by Mews Photosetting, Beckenham, Kent
Printed in Great Britain by St Edmundsbury Press, Suffolk

ISBN 0 412 75640 4

Apart from any fair dealing for the purposes of research or private study, or criticism or review, as permitted under the UK Copyright Designs and Patents Act, 1988, this publication may not be reproduced, stored, or transmitted, in any form or by any means, without the prior permission in writing of the publishers, or in the case of reprographic reproduction only in accordance with the terms of the licences issued by the Copyright Licensing Agency in the UK, or in accordance with the terms of licences issued by the appropriate Reproduction Rights Organization outside the UK. Enquiries concerning reproduction outside the terms stated here should be sent to the publishers at the London address printed on this page.

The publisher makes no representation, express or implied, with regard to the accuracy of the information contained in this book and cannot accept any legal responsibility or liability for any errors or omissions that may be made.

A catalogue record for this book is available from the British Library

Library of Congress Cataloging-in-Publication Data available

∞ Printed on permanent acid-free text paper, manufactured in accordance with ANSI/NISO Z39.48-1992 and ANSI/NISO Z39.48-1984 (Permanence of Paper).

Contents

Preface vi

1. Cell physiology — 1
2. Muscle — 13
3. Peripheral neurophysiology — 32
4. Central neurophysiology — 41
5. Sensory physiology — 51
6. Autonomic nervous system — 63
7. Gastrointestinal physiology — 78
8. Cardiovascular physiology — 91
9. Respiratory physiology — 111
10. Renal physiology — 128
11. Endocrinology — 139
12. Reproductive physiology — 155
13. Answers — 166

Preface

This book contains a selection of multi-choice questions which have been used for assessment in second-year science courses in Physiology at Monash University over many years. We feel that they represent a useful bank of multiple choice questions, which can be used by students studying Physiology as part of a Science degree, a Medical degree, or as part of paramedical or preclinical training. The material covered in any particular Physiology course, from year to year and from place to place, depends on the individual academic teacher. It is likely that this book will contain questions on areas that have not been covered in a particular course in a particular year. Therefore, these questions should not be interpreted to represent a syllabus for any particular course in Physiology.

The format of the questions is that students are required to choose the 'best' of the four options. Under the conditions that the questions were devised and used, students were encouraged to attempt all questions in a particular test or examination, and were not penalized for wrong answers. Many of the questions have been devised and refined by members of the staff of the Physiology Department; we have acted mainly as editors. Answers are given for all of the multiple choice questions at the end of the book.

We are indebted to Ms Kathleen Torkko for the initial editorial work and typesetting.

Every effort has been made to ensure the accuracy of the answers provided. We would appreciate being notified of any errors or discrepancies and any comments for improving future editions.

Chris Browne and Tony Luff
Department of Physiology,
Monash University,
Clayton Campus,
Victoria, Australia.
September 1996

1 Cell physiology

QUESTIONS

1 The most plentiful cation in the interstitial fluid is:
(a) sodium.
(b) chloride.
(c) calcium.
(d) potassium.

2 Which one of the following ions is not normally present in physiological saline solutions such as Krebs' solution?
(a) K^+.
(b) Fe^{2+}.
(c) HCO_3^-.
(d) Mg^{2+}.

3 Cell membranes are highly permeable for water because:
(a) there are many specialized protein channels which enable free diffusion of water across membranes.
(b) water is a non-polar molecule.
(c) water is actively transported (pumped) across the cell membrane.
(d) water is a small molecule.

4 The membrane of cells consists of two layers of phospholipid molecules with protein molecules:
(a) sandwiched between them.
(b) spread on the outside.
(c) held in the membrane in a regular array.
(d) held in the membrane but free to move in it.

2 Multiple Choice Questions in Physiology

5 In a nerve cell:
(a) the axon is usually thicker than the dendrites.
(b) the apparatus for protein synthesis is found only in the cell body.
(c) the axons are usually more numerous than the dendrites.
(d) most of the synapses are formed upon the cell body.

6 The end of an axon may be 1 m distant from the cell body. The axonal ending survives because:
(a) proteins in it are broken down and replaced slowly by local synthesis.
(b) proteins are made almost exclusively in the cell body and are transported to the axon terminal at about $30\,\mathrm{m\,s^{-1}}$.
(c) proteins are supplied to the axon terminal by the postsynaptic cell and by surrounding Schwann cells.
(d) soluble proteins are transported down the axon at about $4\,\mathrm{mm\,day^{-1}}$ and membrane-bound proteins at about $400\,\mathrm{mm\,day^{-1}}$.

7 When a peripheral nerve is cut the:
(a) part between the cell body and the cut soon degenerates.
(b) part between the cut and the peripheral receptors or muscles soon degenerates.
(c) cut heals and conduction of impulses is resumed.
(d) nerve regenerates but does not make functional reconnections with muscle or receptors.

8 A 7.5% solution of potassium chloride (molecular weight 75) has:
(a) an osmolarity of 0.2.
(b) a molarity of 10.
(c) a molarity of 0.1.
(d) an osmolarity of 2.

9 What is the approximate osmolarity of a solution containing 0.50 mol of urea, 0.15 mol of NaCl and 0.05 mol of $CaCl_2$ per litre of solution?
(a) 0.70 Osmolar.
(b) 0.20 Osmolar.
(c) 0.95 Osmolar.
(d) 0.30 Osmolar.

10 Which statement is CORRECT?
(a) Tonicity can never be higher than osmolarity.
(b) Osmolarity can never be higher than tonicity.
(c) Tonicity and osmolarity are not equal at a semipermeable membrane.
(d) Tonicity and osmolarity are equal at a selectively permeable membrane.

11 Osmotic pressure:
(a) is produced without any actual movement of water molecules across a membrane.
(b) is opposite in direction to the concentration gradient of total solutes across a membrane.
(c) is generated by ions and small molecules that try to diffuse across a membrane.
(d) occurs only at a semipermeable membrane.

12 Which one of the following solutions is hypotonic but hyperosmotic for a mammalian red blood cell?
(a) 0.12 M NaCl + 0.9 M urea.
(b) 0.12 M NaCl + 0.9 M sucrose.
(c) 0.12 M $CaCl_2$ + 0.9 M urea.
(d) 0.12 M Na_2SO_4 + 0.9 M propylene glycol.

13 A solution containing 0.1 M NaCl plus 0.28 M urea will make red blood cells immersed in it:
(a) shrink and remain crenated.
(b) swell and burst.
(c) swell at first and then shrink.
(d) shrink at first and then swell.

14 When placed in a slightly hypotonic solution of NaCl, mammalian red blood cells do NOT haemolyse because:
(a) water leaves the cells faster than it enters.
(b) the cells can change shape to accommodate some extra water.
(c) the cell membrane is rigid.
(d) exchange of intracellular K^+ for extracellular Na^+ rapidly produces ionic equilibrium.

15 A 1 M solution of urea will make red blood cells immersed in it:
(a) shrink and then swell but not burst.
(b) shrink and then swell and burst.
(c) shrink and remain crenated.
(d) swell and burst.

16 Glycerol penetrates the red blood cell membrane rather slowly. Which one of the following will happen when red blood cells are suspended in a 1 M solution of glycerol? They will:
(a) immediately undergo haemolysis.
(b) shrink, becoming permanently crenated.
(c) swell first and then shrink to become permanently crenated.
(d) shrink first and then swell and haemolyse.

17 An increased fragility of red blood cells would be indicated by:
(a) their earlier bursting in a hypertonic solution.
(b) a change from translucency to transparency in a slightly hypotonic solution.
(c) a change from translucency to transparency in a very hypotonic solution.
(d) their later bursting in a hypotonic solution.

18 Red blood cells are suspended in solutions containing various concentrations of a freely soluble solute if the:
(a) turbid suspension does not clear in a saturated solution, then the solute is unable to cross the cell membrane.
(b) turbid suspension does clear in a weak solution, then the solute is able to cross the cell membrane.
(c) turbid suspension does clear in a strong solution, then the solute is unable to cross the cell membrane.
(d) clear suspension becomes turbid in a strong solution, then the solute is able to cross the cell membrane.

19 When an excitable cell is in the resting state the:
(a) membrane is more permeable to K^+ than to small, lipid-soluble molecules.
(b) membrane is more permeable to K^+ than to Na^+.
(c) membrane is completely impermeable to Cl^-.
(d) Na^+ pump is turned off.

20 In a resting axon, the active transport of Na^+:
(a) is the immediate cause of the resting potential.
(b) is associated with equal but opposite active transport of K^+.
(c) is stimulated by cardiac glycosides such as ouabain.
(d) just balances the inward diffusion of Na^+.

21 The resting membrane potential in nerve cells is thought to:
(a) be due to an ionic equilibrium described by the Nernst equation.
(b) be due to the outward pumping of three ions of sodium in exchange for only two ions of potassium.
(c) be due to a steady-state condition in which energy is used for pumping sodium and potassium ions across the membrane.
(d) distinguish them from non-signalling cells, for the latter do not usually have resting membrane potentials.

22 The resting membrane potential is mainly due to:
(a) diffusion of some Na^+ out of the cell.
(b) diffusion of some Cl^- out of the cell.
(c) diffusion of some K^+ out of the cell.
(d) active pumping of K^+ out of the cell.

23 Which statement about the equilibrium potentials for Na^+ and K^+ (E_{Na} and E_K) is INCORRECT?
(a) E_{Na} is about $+60\,mV$.
(b) E_{Na} is very close to $0\,mV$.
(c) E_K is about $-90\,mV$.
(d) E_K is somewhat more negative than the resting membrane potential.

24 Cells are said to be in a steady state (as opposed to equilibrium) when:
(a) no expenditure of energy is required to maintain the distribution of ions.
(b) the net flux of cations is equal but opposite to the net flux of anions.
(c) there is no flux of water or any cation or anion.
(d) the resting membrane potential equals the K^+ equilibrium potential minus the Na^+ equilibrium potential.

25 In an excitable cell at rest, the net driving force on intracellular cations is:
(a) Na^+ down its concentration gradient and up its electric gradient.
(b) K^+ down its concentration gradient and down its electric gradient.
(c) Na^+ up its concentration gradient and up its electric gradient.
(d) K^+ up its concentration gradient and up its electric gradient.

26 The sodium pump in the nerve membrane:
(a) is the immediate cause of the negative polarity inside the nerve.
(b) steadily lowers the sodium concentration inside a resting nerve.
(c) is accelerated by a fall in membrane potential.
(d) is accelerated by a rise in internal sodium concentration.

27 The active extrusion of Na⁺ from cells:
(a) is stimulated by the cardiac glycoside ouabain.
(b) depends directly on the presence of Ca^{2+} in the extracellular fluid.
(c) can never make any contribution to the resting membrane potential.
(d) depends on the presence of K^+ in the extracellular fluid.

28 In an axon, the sodium/potassium pump:
(a) steadily decreases the internal concentration of potassium.
(b) repolarizes the membrane after an action potential.
(c) just balances the inward diffusion of sodium.
(d) ensures that the membrane will be negative inside.

29 Which one of the following is likely to occur immediately after blocking the sodium pump in a large excitable cell?
(a) Reduction of the resting membrane potential to zero within a few seconds.
(b) A barely detectable depolarization of a few millivolts.
(c) Immediate reversal of the sodium equilibrium potential.
(d) A marked reduction in the rate of repolarization of the action potential.

30 Doubling the K⁺ concentration outside a nerve fibre causes:
(a) inhibition of the sodium pump.
(b) a decrease in excitability.
(c) some depolarization.
(d) loss of intracellular Cl^-.

31 If there is more K⁺ inside an axon and more Na⁺ outside, it follows that the membrane:
(a) will be positive on the inside.
(b) potential can be predicted from knowledge of the concentration of Na^+ and K^+ on both sides of the membrane.
(c) potential cannot be predicted from the information given.
(d) will be negative on the inside.

32 When there is more K⁺ inside than outside an axon and more Na⁺ outside than inside, the membrane potential must always be:
(a) negative on the inside.
(b) positive on the inside if sodium permeability is greater than potassium permeability.
(c) positive or negative on the inside depending on the concentration gradients of these ions.
(d) negative on the inside provided that potassium permeability is less than sodium permeability.

33 The permeability of a cell membrane to ions that are diffusing across the membrane into the cell is:
(a) reduced if ions are also diffusing out of the cell.
(b) reduced if ions are being actively pumped out of the cell.
(c) reduced if other ions are also diffusing into the cell.
(d) unaffected by (a), (b) or (c) above.

34 If an anode maintains a hyperpolarization of 20 mV in a nerve membrane at a point (X) directly below it and of 5 mV at a point (Y) 6 mm away, what degree of hyperpolarization would be needed at X or Y to be hyperpolarized by 10 mV?
(a) 25 mV.
(b) 30 mV.
(c) 40 mV.
(d) 35 mV.

35 The Puffer-fish poison, tetrodotoxin:
(a) inhibits the Na^+ pump.
(b) blocks the increase in Na^+ permeability during the depolarization phase of the nerve impulse.
(c) blocks the synthesis of ATP.
(d) causes a large increase in Ca^{2+} permeability.

36 When an axon is stimulated to threshold the:
(a) outward K^+ current exceeds the inward Na^+ current.
(b) inward K^+ current exceeds the outward Na^+ current.
(c) outward Na^+ current exceeds the inward K^+ current.
(d) inward Na^+ current exceeds the outward K^+ current.

37 The all-or-nothing nature of the nerve impulse is due to the permeability to Na^+ increasing with:
(a) hyperpolarization and Na^+ entry producing further depolarization.
(b) depolarization and Na^+ entry producing further depolarization.
(c) depolarization and Na^+ entry producing further hyperpolarization.
(d) hyperpolarization and Na^+ entry producing further hyperpolarization.

38 During a nerve action potential:
(a) Na^+ enters the axon and K^+ leaves it.
(b) the membrane is hyperpolarized.
(c) K^+ enters the axon and Na^+ leaves it.
(d) acetylcholine depolarizes the nerve membrane.

39 At the peak of an action potential, the:
(a) net membrane current falls to zero.
(b) internal sodium concentration approximates to that outside the axon.
(c) membrane is subjected to the largest voltage gradient that it experiences.
(d) sodium equilibrium potential is reached.

40 During the passage of a nerve impulse:
(a) sodium enters the axon and raises the concentration in the axoplasm to be nearly equal to the external sodium concentration.
(b) the sodium that has entered is pumped out again so that the next impulse can be propagated.
(c) so little sodium enters the axon that the membrane potential is hardly affected.
(d) the amount of sodium that enters is limited by inactivation of the sodium permeability.

41 An action potential travels along an axon by:
(a) releasing acetylcholine to stimulate the membrane ahead.
(b) causing a flow of current across the myelin sheath.
(c) causing a flow of current that hyperpolarizes the axon ahead.
(d) causing a flow of current that makes the inside of the axon ahead less negative.

42 In an axon carrying an action potential at a velocity of $25\,\text{m}\,\text{s}^{-1}$, the length of the active region is 30 mm. What is the duration of the action potential at a point on the axon?
(a) 0.83 ms.
(b) 1.2 ms.
(c) 0.75 ms.
(d) 8.3 ms.

43 The length of axon occupied by a nerve impulse at an instant of time:
(a) is greater in smaller axons.
(b) increases with the strength of the electrical stimulus that started it.
(c) is decreased in axons of low threshold.
(d) increases with conduction velocity and with duration of the impulse.

44 When an action potential reaches the end of a nerve fibre, it does not return along the fibre because:
(a) nerve fibres are capable of conducting in one direction only.
(b) too much sodium has entered the nerve fibre.
(c) the end of the nerve is inexcitable.
(d) inactivation of the voltage-dependent increase in sodium permeability occurs.

45 When an electric stimulus applied to an axon is slightly too small to start an action potential:
(a) the subsequent outward diffusion of positive ions exceeds the inward diffusion of positive ions.
(b) the resting membrane potential is restored by the activity of the sodium/potassium pump.
(c) no depolarization is produced.
(d) depolarization increases sodium permeability, which makes the inside of the axon more negative.

46 A nerve trunk with a wide spectrum of fibre sizes gives a compound action potential in which the later deflections are due to fibres of:
(a) low threshold and high conduction velocity.
(b) low conduction velocity and high threshold.
(c) large diameter and low threshold.
(d) low conduction velocity and low threshold.

47 In a nerve trunk:
(a) an axon is stimulated to threshold when outward current exceeds inward current.
(b) smaller axons are stimulated by a smaller change of membrane potential than large axons.
(c) threshold is decreased by the depolarization remaining just after the passage of a previous nerve impulse.
(d) the lower apparent threshold of large axons is mainly due to their smaller longitudinal resistance.

48 If the rise in sodium permeability were not inactivated at the peak of an action potential:
(a) the axon membrane would be positively charged on the inside for a prolonged period.
(b) action potentials would be able to follow each other more closely than usual because there would be no absolute refractory period.
(c) the electrical potential of the inside of the axon would rise to $+90\,mV$.
(d) the sodium pump would gradually restore the resting membrane potential.

49 The repolarizing phase of the action potential is:
(a) due to a delayed increase in the ratio of the Na^+ permeability to the K^+ permeability of the excitable membrane.
(b) due to increased rate of extrusion of Na^+ by the sodium pump.
(c) associated with an increased rate of K^+ efflux.
(d) due to a delayed increase in the Na^+ conductance of the excitable membrane.

50 After sodium permeability is inactivated at the peak of a nerve impulse, the membrane potential will recover the resting value:
(a) when the sodium/potassium pump has extruded the sodium ions that have entered.
(b) as positive ions diffuse out of the axon.
(c) at the beginning of the relative refractory period.
(d) when potassium ions diffuse into the axon.

51 When a nerve trunk containing both large and small axons is stimulated electrically, small shocks stimulate:
(a) only the smaller axons because their threshold is smaller.
(b) only the larger axons because their internal resistance is smaller.
(c) only the larger axons because their internal resistance is larger.
(d) certain axons whose membranes require a smaller depolarization in order to give an action potential.

52 When two electrodes applied to a stimulated nerve record a diphasic action potential, the second phase is due to:
(a) impulses reaching the electrode furthest from the point of stimulation.
(b) recovery processes in the nerve.
(c) impulses being conducted in both directions away from the point of stimulation.
(d) local circuit current.

53 When two electrical stimuli 10 ms apart are applied to a motor nerve the:
(a) muscle fibres innervated give larger action potentials in response to the second stimulus.
(b) muscle fibres innervated give no action potentials.
(c) motor nerve does not respond to the second stimulus because it is still in the absolute refractory period.
(d) concentration of free calcium in the muscle fibres innervated is highest after the second stimulus.

Cell physiology

54 In the relative refractory period of a nerve the:
(a) inward movement of K^+ raises the threshold.
(b) inward movement of K^+ lowers the threshold.
(c) outward movement of K^+ raises the threshold.
(d) outward movement of K^+ lowers the threshold.

55 In the absolute refractory period of a nerve the:
(a) Na^+ permeability fails to rise with depolarization.
(b) membrane resistance is higher than in resting nerve.
(c) membrane is hyperpolarized.
(d) K^+ permeability is decreased.

56 When a nerve trunk is stimulated, and the responses recorded 5 cm away, the smaller axons give:
(a) a late response because they require a stronger stimulus.
(b) an earlier response because they have a high internal resistance.
(c) a late response because the stimulus current is conducted more slowly.
(d) a late response because their action potentials are propagated more slowly.

57 Which statement about G_m (the conductance of unit area of membrane) is INCORRECT?
(a) $G_m = C_m \times \tau_m$ where C_m is the capacitance of unit area of cell membrane and τ_m is the membrane time constant.
(b) G_m is related to membrane permeability for ions.
(c) $G_m = G_{Na} + G_K + G_{Cl}$
(d) $G_m = 1/R_m$, where R_m is the resistance of unit area of cell membrane.

58 The velocity of conduction of the nerve impulse depends on the:
(a) duration of the refractory period.
(b) strength of stimulation.
(c) direction of conduction.
(d) diameter of the nerve fibre.

59 If an axon forms two branches which are each one-quarter of the diameter of the parent axon, the parent axon conducts impulses:
(a) twice as fast as the branches if all of the axons are myelinated.
(b) as fast as the branches if none of the axons are myelinated.
(c) at twice the frequency of the branches if all the axons are myelinated.
(d) four times faster than the branches if none of the axons is myelinated.

60   If a myelinated nerve fibre whose diameter was 10 μm had a conduction velocity of 60 m s^{-1}, what would you expect the diameter to be of a fibre having a conduction velocity of 120 m s^{-1}?
(a) 2 μm.
(b) 6 μm.
(c) 20 μm.
(d) 60 μm.

2 Muscle

QUESTIONS

1 Miniature endplate potentials:
(a) are 40–140 mV in amplitude.
(b) initiate contractions in single muscle fibres.
(c) occur at regular intervals in small muscles.
(d) are caused by small amounts of acetylcholine.

2 Miniature endplate potentials, which occur spontaneously at motor endplates, are due to:
(a) the random firing of action potentials in nerve terminals.
(b) the diffusion of single molecules of acetylcholine across the membrane of the nerve terminal.
(c) random 'noise' which is generated in the nerve terminal due to its low electrical resistance.
(d) the simultaneous release of several thousand molecules of acetylcholine.

3 Which statement does NOT apply to the synthesis of acetylcholine in motor nerve terminals?
(a) Synthesis depends on the uptake of choline by the membrane of the nerve terminal.
(b) Acetylcholine is synthesized within the synaptic vesicles.
(c) Synthesis depends on the presence of ATP.
(d) The rate of synthesis increases when the nerve terminal is stimulated.

4 Following stimulation of the motor nerve, the action potential recorded at an endplate of a skeletal muscle fibre differs from the action potential recorded at other parts of the fibre in that the action potential recorded at the endplate:
(a) has a different shape due to the relatively high permeabilities of the membrane to both Na^+ and K^+.
(b) has a different shape due to the diffusion of charged molecules of the transmitter substance through the membrane.
(c) has a larger amplitude.
(d) is briefer.

5 Transmission at the neuromuscular junction is caused by:
(a) electrical spread of excitation due to the cable properties of the nerve and muscle fibres.
(b) release of Ca^{2+} ions from presynaptic vesicles.
(c) release of a chemical transmitter from the nerve terminals.
(d) the protoplasmic continuity between nerve and muscle fibres.

6 The initial depolarization of the endplate potential is caused by:
(a) an inward flow of potassium ions.
(b) the passive cable properties of muscle fibres.
(c) a sudden increase in the postsynaptic membrane impedance.
(d) an inward flow of sodium ions.

7 The release of acetylcholine from the skeletal neuromuscular junction:
(a) is dependent on the presence of Ca^{2+} in the medium surrounding the nerve terminal.
(b) results in a decrease in the permeability of the postsynaptic membrane to both Na^+ and K^+.
(c) leads to the development of an endplate potential in the presynaptic cell.
(d) is potentiated by the presence of Mg^{2+} in the medium surrounding the nerve terminal.

8 At skeletal neuromuscular junctions released transmitter is inactivated largely by:
(a) diffusion away from receptor sites.
(b) spontaneous breakdown into inert compounds.
(c) enzymatic breakdown.
(d) reabsorption into nerve terminals.

Muscle

9 Acetylcholine causes depolarization of the endplate region of skeletal muscles because it:
(a) is positively charged and enters the cell, as does Na^+ during its action potential.
(b) causes an increase in conductance for Na^+ ions only.
(c) causes an increase in conductance for Na^+, K^+ and Ca^{2+}.
(d) causes an increase in conductance for both cations and anions.

10 At all skeletal neuromuscular junctions, the duration of transmitter action is largely determined by:
(a) diffusion away from its release site.
(b) breakdown by monoamine oxidase (MAO).
(c) uptake into nerve terminals.
(d) hydrolysis, catalysed by choline esterase.

11 In a low calcium, high magnesium environment, transmission at the skeletal neuromuscular junction is depressed because:
(a) release of acetylcholine is decreased.
(b) the synthesis of acetylcholine is decreased.
(c) the number of molecules in each quantum of acetylcholine is reduced.
(d) magnesium has a curare-like action on the skeletal muscle membrane.

12 The action of curare at the skeletal neuromuscular junction is due to the:
(a) blockage of the acetylcholine receptors in the postsynaptic membrane and hence a reduction in the amplitude of the endplate potential.
(b) interference with the entry of calcium into the nerve terminals.
(c) reduction in the amplitude of the endplate potentials by partially blocking the passage of action potentials in the nerve in the region of the neuromuscular junction.
(d) partial blockage of transmission of the action potential down the tubules of the transverse tubular system, thereby reducing the amount of tension the muscle can produce.

13 The arrival of an action potential at the nerve endplate of a skeletal muscle fibre:
(a) always causes the generation of an action potential in the muscle fibre by means of direct electrical coupling between the pre- and postsynaptic membranes.
(b) gives rise to an endplate potential of sufficient amplitude to generate an action potential in the muscle fibre.
(c) causes release of acetylcholine from the postsynaptic cell which in turn gives rise to an action potential in the presynaptic cell.
(d) will only give rise to an action potential in the muscle fibre if enough action potentials arrive at the nerve terminal to produce a sufficiently large endplate potential.

14 An endplate potential at the skeletal neuromuscular junction:
(a) is the result of current flow across the muscle membrane, directly generated by the action potential invading the nerve terminal.
(b) would be reduced by substances that inhibit the enzyme choline esterase.
(c) is the result of an increase in the conductance for cations of the muscle endplate region.
(d) is unaffected by reduction of Na^+ concentration in the surrounding medium.

15 Which statement does NOT apply to the synthesis of acetylcholine in motor nerve terminals?
(a) Acetylcholine is synthesized in the cytosol.
(b) Synthesis depends on the active uptake of choline by the nerve terminal membrane.
(c) Synthesis depends on the enzyme choline esterase.
(d) Synthesis involves acetyl-coenzyme A.

16 At skeletal neuromuscular junctions, the action of acetylcholine is brief because:
(a) there is a high concentration of the enzyme choline acetylase in the endplate region.
(b) acetylcholine is taken up into nerve terminals.
(c) the area of the muscle membrane occupied by receptors is small.
(d) acetylcholine is rapidly broken down into inactive components.

17 In a normal, innervated skeletal muscle fibre acetylcholine receptors are found:
(a) concentrated in the muscle fibre membrane close to the nerve terminal.
(b) lining the tubules of the transverse tubular system.
(c) on the presynaptic membrane.
(d) distributed along the whole length of the surface membrane of the muscle fibre.

18 Excitation–contraction coupling in skeletal muscle is thought to involve:
(a) depolarization of the transverse (T) tubules.
(b) a large influx of Ca^{2+} from the extracellular space.
(c) inactivation of the sodium pump.
(d) hyperpolarization of the Z band.

19 The ion most directly involved in excitation–contraction coupling in skeletal muscle is:
(a) Na^+.
(b) Cl^-.
(c) Ca^{2+}.
(d) K^+.

20 Which statement is INCORRECT?
(a) Calcium ions provide the link between excitation and contraction in all types of muscles.
(b) Calcium ion concentration in the sarcoplasm of a resting muscle fibre is very low.
(c) Increasing extracellular calcium triggers the contraction cycle in skeletal muscle.
(d) Calcium ions play a role in the mechanism of release of transmitter at the neuromuscular junction.

21 For some time after calcium is removed from the fluid bathing an isolated skeletal muscle, the fibres continue to contract in response to direct stimulation. Taken together with other evidence, this observation shows that:
(a) calcium is not involved in excitation–contraction coupling.
(b) excitation is not dependent on an action potential mechanism.
(c) the calcium involved in excitation–contraction coupling must be released from intracellular stores.
(d) release of acetylcholine by the nerve terminal does not require extracellular Ca^{2+}.

22 The conduction of excitation down the transverse tubules of skeletal muscle fibres:
(a) is a passive process dependent on the passive membrane properties of the transverse tubule.
(b) is a regenerative process not unlike that in the surface membrane.
(c) can be prevented by the presence of curare.
(d) is not affected by temperature.

23 In resting skeletal muscle the free calcium ion concentration is low because:
(a) the outer cell membrane is impermeable to calcium in the resting state.
(b) calcium is bound by actomyosin during the hydrolysis of ATP.
(c) it is actively pumped back into the sarcoplasmic reticulum.
(d) all available calcium is used up during the contraction cycle.

24 The major known function of the transverse tubular system of skeletal muscle fibres is to:
(a) cause mechanically the fibre to lengthen after completion of a contraction.
(b) inactivate transmitter.
(c) convey electrical excitation.
(d) provide a harness for myofilaments to transmit their tension.

25 The myosin filaments of skeletal muscle are:
(a) thinner than the actin filaments.
(b) attached to the triads.
(c) attached to the Z line.
(d) found only in the A band.

26 The interaction between actin and myosin in mammalian skeletal muscle is controlled by the:
(a) binding of calcium to the myosin.
(b) action of calcium within the head region of the myosin molecule.
(c) specific regulator proteins located on the actin filament.
(d) presence of troponin and tropomyosin on the thick myosin filament.

27 All the following are true of the transverse tubular system (or T-system) of skeletal muscle EXCEPT it:
(a) forms the outer components of the structures known as 'Triads'.
(b) is seen at the Z line in the skeletal muscle of lower vertebrates such as the frog.
(c) is continuous with the sarcolemma (surface membrane).
(d) forms an electrical path for the conduction of excitation into the interior of a muscle fibre.

28 In striated muscle:
(a) all ATP must be removed to prevent the actomyosin complex from being broken down.
(b) each cross-bridge contributes only once to the generation of force.
(c) myosin will only complex with ATP in the presence of magnesium ions.
(d) calcium acts to facilitate the inhibitory action of the troponin–tropomyosin complex.

29 If the optimum length (L_0) of a skeletal muscle is 100%, then in changing from a length of 120% L_0 to 80% L_0 the:
(a) A band remains unchanged and the I band and H zone decrease in length.
(b) A band increases and the I band decreases in length.
(c) sarcomere length increases.
(d) passive tension of the muscle increases.

30 The regulatory proteins tropomyosin and troponin:
(a) are located along the helically coiled myosin molecule.
(b) inhibit the active sites on the actin molecule.
(c) determine the cycle rate of an individual cross-bridge.
(d) split ATP during contraction.

31 Cross-bridges between actin and myosin filaments of skeletal muscle:
(a) occur mainly near the Z line.
(b) occur solely in the A band.
(c) are responsible for lengthening the fibres.
(d) serve principally to damp down the tension produced during a contraction.

32 In the cross-bridge cycle, binding of ATP immediately precedes:
(a) removal of the inhibitory influence of tropomyosin and troponin.
(b) the formation of the actomyosin complex prior to the 'power stroke'.
(c) rapid dissociation of the actomyosin complex.
(d) the removal of calcium from the regulator protein troponin.

33 A single mammalian skeletal muscle myofibril:
(a) consists of many sarcomeres in parallel.
(b) is 2–3 µm long.
(c) consists of many myofibrils and nuclei enclosed by the sarcolemma.
(d) is enclosed by a sleeve of sarcoplasmic reticulum and encircled at the A/I boundary by the transverse tubular system.

34 **The state of rigor mortis in an animal:**
(a) is associated with the inhibitory influence of the troponin–tropomyosin complex on the contraction cycle.
(b) is the result of natural processes of decay which act to break down the contractile proteins.
(c) commences when the muscle's reserves of ATP are used up.
(d) is signalled by the inability of the myosin heads, once they are detached, from reattaching to new sites on the thin filament.

35 **Force recorded from an isolated skeletal muscle preparation will be increased by:**
(a) initiating the contraction after the muscle has been shortened.
(b) initiating the contraction when the muscle is in a condition such that the Z lines lie close to each other.
(c) increasing the series elasticity.
(d) giving two closely spaced stimuli instead of a single stimulus.

36 **Some skeletal muscles contract more quickly than others because:**
(a) they depend entirely on glycolytic metabolism as a source of energy.
(b) they tend to have a lower rate of release of calcium ions during the contraction cycle.
(c) they are composed exclusively of small fatigue-resistant muscle fibres.
(d) the rate of cross-bridge detachment is higher.

37 **Tension recorded from an isolated skeletal muscle preparation will be increased by:**
(a) initiating the contraction when the muscle is in a condition such that the Z lines lie as close to each other as possible.
(b) increasing the series elasticity.
(c) giving two stimuli 5 ms apart instead of a single stimulus.
(d) giving two stimuli 0.5 ms apart instead of a single stimulus.

38 **Prolonged tetanic stimulation of the sciatic nerve of a toad sciatic–gastrocnemius preparation usually causes fatigue:**
(a) in the nerve fibres due to depletion of K^+ reserves.
(b) at the neuromuscular junction (shown by stimulating muscle directly).
(c) in the muscle fibres (shown by the build-up of ATP).
(d) in the muscle fibres (shown by their sensitivity to acetylcholine).

39 A motor unit:
(a) consists of all the muscles acting about the same joint.
(b) will progressively increase its contractile force as the strength of the stimulus to the nerve supply of the muscle is increased.
(c) will progressively increase its contractile force as the rate of stimulation of the muscle nerve is increased.
(d) comprises at least 10% of the total number of fibres in a muscle.

40 A muscle develops its maximal tension:
(a) when a single supramaximal stimulus is applied to the muscle nerve.
(b) at a length corresponding to the maximum as measured in the body.
(c) when there is proportionately little overlap between the thick and thin filaments of sarcomeres.
(d) when there is maximal overlap between thick and thin filaments.

41 The contraction of a whole skeletal muscle may be increased in a smooth (graded) fashion by means of:
(a) an increase in the amplitude of the action potential in a single nerve fibre leading to a prolonged activation of contractile elements.
(b) an increase in the number of nerve fibres activated (recruitment).
(c) an increase in the number of muscle fibres activated by a single nerve fibre (recruitment).
(d) a decrease in the frequency of activation of a single nerve fibre leading to a summation of contraction.

42 In skeletal muscle the twitch tension would be as big as the tetanic tension if:
(a) the muscle was stimulated sufficiently strongly to engage all motoneurones.
(b) each nerve impulse activated muscle fibres along their entire length.
(c) in response to a single action potential muscle fibres could stretch their tendinous connections fast enough to develop in them the full tension generated in sarcomeres.
(d) the intrinsic speed of shortening of muscle fibres was sufficiently high.

43 Summation of muscle contraction occurs when:
(a) the calcium has been pumped back into the sarcoplasmic reticulum and the muscle is ready to contract again.
(b) the second stimulus is given after the peak of the contraction produced by the first stimulus.
(c) the contraction following the second stimulus does not have to completely re-stretch the series elastic element.
(d) some potentiation of neuromuscular transmission is observed.

44 A muscle which in the adult animal is of the slowly contracting variety:
(a) was able to contract more rapidly while in its embryonic form.
(b) will remain slow even after its nerve has been cut and the nerve from a fast muscle been allowed to grow into it.
(c) probably remains slow because of the combined influences of impulse traffic and substances secreted by the motoneurones.
(d) is characterized by its susceptibility to fatigue in response to prolonged repetitive stimulation.

45 Graded contraction of a muscle, initiated reflexly:
(a) is achieved by controlling the number of muscle fibres contracting in a single motor unit.
(b) recruits the small motor units before the large ones.
(c) is only possible by altering the number of active motor units.
(d) is dependent on central inhibitory mechanisms.

46 The growth of a limb muscle is favoured by all the following EXCEPT:
(a) increased work due to increased nerve activity.
(b) rest permitted by lack of nerve activity.
(c) male sex hormones.
(d) inactivation of other muscles that normally have a similar action within the same limb.

47 During early development:
(a) muscle contraction cannot occur until innervation by motor nerves is complete.
(b) there is a period during which single muscle fibres may have more than one motor nerve terminal.
(c) muscle tends, overall, to have a briefer contraction time.
(d) the myoblast is the cell type destined to represent the neuromuscular junction of the mature muscle cell.

48 Summation of contractions in skeletal muscle:
(a) gives rise to the staircase phenomenon.
(b) is proportional to the number of motor units activated.
(c) depends on the long refractory period of skeletal muscle.
(d) is an important mechanism in the grading of contraction.

49 In normal use a skeletal muscle is extended by the action of:
(a) repulsive forces between the thick and thin filaments.
(b) the elastic nature of the sarcolemma.
(c) its series elastic element.
(d) an appropriate antagonist muscle.

50 Summation of contraction in single muscle fibres is possible because:
(a) during a twitch the duration of activation of the contractile machinery is not long enough to permit complete shortening of sarcomeres.
(b) during a twitch none of the myofibrils is activated.
(c) during a single contraction the amount of available ATP is limiting.
(d) parallel elastic components exert a frictional resistance on the contraction.

51 In the toad sciatic–gastrocnemius preparation used in the practical class, 'recruitment' depended on greater:
(a) stimulus voltages being able to stimulate muscle fibres of higher threshold.
(b) stimulus voltages being able to stimulate nerve fibres of higher threshold.
(c) stimulation frequency leading to depolarization of more nerve fibres.
(d) stimulation frequency leading to longer lasting stretch of the series elastic compliance.

52 In skeletal muscle a motor unit consists of:
(a) all the muscle fibres within a single connective tissue bundle.
(b) all the motor and sensory nerves supplying a single muscle fibre.
(c) all the muscle fibres having the same threshold for electrical stimulation.
(d) a motor nerve fibre and all the muscle fibres it supplies.

53 During isometric contraction in skeletal muscle:
(a) the true internal tension at the level of the sarcomeres is never realized because of the presence of external passive tension.
(b) tension at the level of the sarcomeres is always less than that in the tendon because the tendon is being stretched.
(c) each cross-bridge contributes only once during the contraction.
(d) cross-bridges in the two halves of each sarcomere pull in opposite directions.

54 Those skeletal muscles involved in finely controlled movements:
(a) have relatively long fibres and short tendons.
(b) have motor units consisting of relatively few muscle fibres.
(c) are innervated by motoneurones whose cell bodies are located in the brain.
(d) consist of muscle fibres which are multiply innervated.

55 Skeletal muscle hypertrophy is due primarily to:
(a) an increase in the number of muscle fibres.
(b) an increase in diameter of the existing fibres.
(c) an increase in the length of the existing fibres.
(d) a relative increase in the myofibrillar proteins at the expense of the sarcoplasmic reticulum and mitochondria.

56 Summation of muscular contraction depends on:
(a) the stimulus being less than maximal.
(b) there being an interval of more than 500 ms between contractions.
(c) the presence of a series elastic component in the muscle.
(d) increased efficiency of the neuromuscular junction.

57 In the practical class, the force produced by the toad gastrocnemius muscle when the sciatic nerve was stimulated electrically was recorded by the:
(a) tension in the muscle moving the pen of the recorder.
(b) pen recorder measuring the electrical response of the muscle.
(c) action potential acting on a strain gauge.
(d) pen recorder measuring a change of resistance in a strain gauge attached to the muscle.

58 During isometric recording of a muscle contraction:
(a) the load on the muscle is kept constant and the amount of shortening is measured.
(b) the length of the muscle is held constant and the total tension measured.
(c) active tension can only be recorded when the level of passive tension is exceeded.
(d) active tension at a muscle length of 150% L_0 will exceed that at 110% L_0.

59 The connective tissue found around skeletal muscle fibres, together with the sarcolemma:
(a) contributes to the development of active tension.
(b) constitutes the parallel elastic element.
(c) permits some internal shortening of the muscle during an isometric contraction.
(d) forms the series elastic element.

60 In the force–velocity relation of skeletal muscle:
(a) there is a direct proportionality between the force developed by the muscle and the speed of shortening.
(b) as the load is increased there is an initial very steep drop in the velocity of shortening followed by a more gradual decline.
(c) the shape of the relation indicates that contracting muscle has no inherent viscosity and can be simply represented as a spring of variable stiffness.
(d) the speed of shortening is independent of the load.

61 In the right hand or descending limb of the active length–tension curve:
(a) tension is at a maximum when the two thin filaments butt up against one another.
(b) the amount of tension produced is determined by the degree of interference between opposing thin filaments.
(c) tension is directly proportional to the amount of overlap between the thick and thin filaments.
(d) tension cannot be measured accurately because of the high level of passive tension.

62 **During an afterloaded isotonic contraction in a skeletal muscle:**
(a) the contractile component shortens while the series elastic component lengthens.
(b) the contractile component shortens while the series elastic component remains unchanged.
(c) both the contractile component and series elastic component shorten.
(d) both the parallel elastic component and series elastic component shorten.

63 **During an isometric contraction in a skeletal muscle:**
(a) a small amount of shortening occurs initially due to the elasticity of the cross-bridges and tendons.
(b) the parallel elastic component will be stretched.
(c) the series elastic component will shorten.
(d) the length of the series elastic component will remain unchanged.

64 **Strength training, involving exercising with relatively high loads and relatively few repetitions, results in:**
(a) the muscle mass remaining unchanged but a conversion of the fast fatiguable fibres to the fast fatigue-resistant fibres.
(b) an increase in muscle mass due to uniform hypertrophy of all fibre types.
(c) muscle fibre hypertrophy due to a preferential increase in sarcoplasmic proteins.
(d) preferential hypertrophy of the fast fatigue-resistant and fast fatiguable fibre types.

65 **Which statement about adult, mammalian motor units is INCORRECT?**
(a) All the muscle fibres in a given motor unit are of the same histochemical type.
(b) Normally, all the muscle fibres in a motor unit are activated when the motoneurone is active.
(c) It is possible for a muscle fibre to be innervated by more than one motoneurone.
(d) A motoneurone may branch repeatedly to innervate a few muscle fibres or several thousand muscle fibres.

66 Which statement is INCORRECT?
(a) The functional unit in muscle, from the point of view of motor control, is the motor unit.
(b) Mammalian muscle fibres commonly receive only one nerve end-plate along their length.
(c) The only way the central nervous system is able to grade the strength of a contraction is to alter the rate of discharge of motoneurones.
(d) Large motoneurones are reflexly less excitable than small ones.

67 The term 'myogenic' refers to a muscle which:
(a) is constantly active as a result of tonic activity in motoneurones.
(b) maintains a steady level of tension from tonic sympathetic drive.
(c) relies exclusively on circulating hormones for the initiation of contractile activity.
(d) is intrinsically active and continues to contract rhythmically even though its motor nerves are not stimulated.

68 During an isotonic contraction:
(a) there is a change in the force of contraction, muscle length being kept constant.
(b) the sarcomeres lengthen.
(c) the muscle length changes while under a constant load.
(d) there is shortening of the A band with no change in the length of the I band.

69 As well as providing a means of attachment of muscles to skeletal structures, tendons are of functional importance because:
(a) during an isotonic contraction their elasticity allows them to propel muscle tension to higher levels.
(b) they ensure that muscle twitch and tetanic tension remain similar.
(c) they are sites for storage of elastic energy.
(d) they co-operate within the cross-bridge mechanism to prevent development within the muscle of dangerously high levels of tension.

70 Shortening speed is higher:
(a) when the muscle bears larger loads.
(b) in motor units with larger innervation ratios.
(c) in muscles with longer muscle fibres.
(d) in postural muscle, compared with muscle involved in fine manipulative movements.

71 During a maintained isometric contraction:
(a) contracting muscle fibres are unable to shorten and therefore are unable to develop their full tension.
(b) contracting muscle fibres shorten progressively more slowly as the tension in the stretched tendons rises.
(c) the tension generated by muscle fibres which rely only on oxidative metabolism will progressively decline due to depletion of metabolic stores.
(d) peak tension levels reached will be less than during an isotonic contraction provided the contraction speed is high enough.

72 The tension developed by a muscle fibre will increase:
(a) if more contractile material is packed in parallel.
(b) when it has more sarcomeres in series.
(c) when it has longer tendons.
(d) when the actomyosin ATPase activity is raised.

73 Mammalian skeletal muscle fibres can be divided into two main types. Which statement is INCORRECT?
(a) Fast-twitch fibres have a relatively short isometric twitch and fast speed of shortening.
(b) Fast-twitch fibres have relatively low myosin ATPase activity and oxidative or glycolytic metabolism.
(c) Slow-twitch fibres have a relatively long isometric twitch and slow speed of shortening.
(d) Slow-twitch fibres have relatively low myosin ATPase activity and oxidative metabolism.

74 All the following statements are true of both skeletal and cardiac muscle, EXCEPT:
(a) the fibres are subdivided into parallel fibrils.
(b) the ultrastructure of the fibres is such that transverse striations can be seen in the electron microscope.
(c) the fibres only contract in response to activity in the nerves which terminate on them.
(d) two types of protein filament can be observed in the electron microscope.

75 The duration of the action potential of human ventricular muscle is usually about:
(a) 25 s.
(b) 25 ms.
(c) 0.25 s.
(d) 2.5 ms.

76 **Cardiac muscle fibres:**
(a) are electrically insulated from each other.
(b) are incapable of contraction in the absence of an intact nerve supply.
(c) have an ionic mechanism for the generation of action potentials which does not depend on the presence of potassium ions.
(d) can excite each other.

77 **Pacemakers are found in all the following EXCEPT:**
(a) duodenal muscle.
(b) uterine muscle.
(c) muscles that move the eye.
(d) sino-atrial node.

78 **A compensatory pause would be exhibited in:**
(a) heart muscle when an electrical stimulus is applied during the refractory period.
(b) heart muscle when an electrical stimulus is applied causing a premature contraction (extrasystole).
(c) skeletal muscle after a series of high frequency stimuli is applied to its motor nerve.
(d) skeletal muscle after an electrical stimulus is applied during the refractory period of the membrane.

79 **Cardiac muscle:**
(a) has a shortening velocity greater than that of skeletal twitch muscle.
(b) is an anatomical syncytium.
(c) is an electrical (functional) syncytium.
(d) has a resting potential that depends mainly on sodium ion distribution.

80 **Conduction of excitation from the atria to the ventricles in the mammalian heart:**
(a) is via the sino-atrial node.
(b) is dependent on the presence of papillary muscles.
(c) can occur anywhere on the boundary between the atria and ventricles.
(d) is restricted to the atrioventricular node.

81 Cells of the sino-atrial node are:
(a) responsible for conducting and delaying the wave of excitation from the atria to the ventricles.
(b) highly specialized sympathetic nerve cells with prolonged action potentials.
(c) specialized cardiac cells incapable of generating action potentials.
(d) autorhythmic and determine the rate of heart beat.

82 In cardiac muscle:
(a) there are paths of low electrical resistance between adjacent muscle fibres.
(b) muscle fibres are electrically insulated from one another but communicate via nerves.
(c) a fused tetanic contraction of heart muscle fibres results from high frequency impulse activity in the innervating nerves.
(d) both sympathetic and parasympathetic nerve fibres supplying the heart exert their influence exclusively by altering excitability of sino-atrial pacemaker cells.

83 The action potential of cardiac muscle:
(a) is associated with a short refractory period.
(b) has a long duration that is comparable with that of a single contraction.
(c) is independent of Na^+ ions.
(d) is a graded phenomenon.

84 Cardiac muscle cells are characterized by having:
(a) very dense sarcoplasmic reticulum and few mitochondria.
(b) specialized cell-to-cell connections which prevent the conduction of an action potential.
(c) several nuclei within each cell.
(d) many mitochondria and relatively little sarcoplasmic reticulum.

85 Smooth muscle:
(a) normally contains the regulator proteins troponin and tropomyosin in the same ratio as skeletal muscle.
(b) has myosin filaments identical in length and packing to those in skeletal muscle.
(c) contains actin filaments and myosin filaments in the approximate ratio of 12:1.
(d) contains troponin but no tropomyosin.

Muscle

86 Smooth muscle has a:
(a) membrane potential that is often unstable.
(b) more extensive sarcoplasmic reticulum than skeletal muscle.
(c) spike discharge rate that is decreased when it is stretched.
(d) myofilament arrangement similar to that found in cardiac muscle.

87 Smooth muscle:
(a) is not electrically excitable.
(b) consists of individual cells which are electrically insulated from each other.
(c) may show myogenic activity.
(d) has characteristic action potentials which are always less than 20 mV in amplitude.

88 In smooth muscle, action potentials are:
(a) only generated when the muscle is stretched.
(b) not conducted between adjacent cells.
(c) always very much smaller than those in skeletal muscle.
(d) conducted between adjacent cells via regions of low electrical resistance.

89 The rising phase of the smooth muscle action potential:
(a) is mainly dependent on an influx of sodium ions.
(b) is accomplished by an influx of calcium ions.
(c) is accomplished by an influx of anions.
(d) requires an influx of potassium ions.

90 Cross-bridge cycling in smooth muscle is regulated by:
(a) calcium binding to troponin in a mechanism similar to that of skeletal muscle.
(b) a calcium–calmodulin complex binding directly to myosin.
(c) activation of a myosin light chain kinase by a calcium–calmodulin complex which phosphorylates the myosin.
(d) calcium activating a myosin light chain kinase leading to phosphorylation of myosin.

91 The active length–tension curve of smooth muscle is:
(a) relatively longer than that of skeletal muscle because of the extensibility of the thick and thin filaments.
(b) about the same as that of skeletal muscle.
(c) relatively longer than that of skeletal muscle because of the lack of organization of the thick and thin filaments.
(d) not dependent on the overlap of thick and thin filaments.

3 Peripheral neurophysiology

QUESTIONS

1 Pacinian corpuscles:
(a) are found only in the skin.
(b) are typically slowly adapting sensory receptors.
(c) respond to high frequency vibration.
(d) have unmyelinated axons.

2 The Pacinian corpuscle:
(a) responds to both the 'on' and 'off' phases of a sustained mechanical prod because it is a slowly adapting receptor.
(b) is found only in non-hairy or glabrous skin.
(c) has its adaptive property conferred to it largely by the lamellated capsule.
(d) has its adaptive property conferred to it only by the properties of the axonal membrane.

3 Muscle spindles:
(a) contain extrafusal fibres.
(b) are activated by Ia fibres.
(c) are supplied by Aα fibres.
(d) are inhibitory to Ib fibres.

4 Muscle spindles:
(a) are thought to signal muscle tension.
(b) provide the prime trigger for locomotion.
(c) are an example of a receptor with access to the cerebral cortex and therefore are implicated in conscious sensation.
(d) represent the receptor of origin for the flexor reflex.

Peripheral neurophysiology

5 Which statement concerning muscle spindles is CORRECT?
(a) They are most commonly located at the muscle–tendon junction.
(b) Afferent volleys in Ia fibres inhibit the homonymous motoneurones.
(c) Secondary sensory endings are commonest on nuclear chain fibres.
(d) The spindle sensory endings are distended by intrafusal relaxation.

6 A muscle spindle will increase its discharge rate:
(a) when the amount of intrafusal shortening consequent upon fusimotor activation is precisely balanced by extrafusal shortening.
(b) during the rising phase of a muscle contraction, as here the contracting extrafusal fibres are pulling directly on the spindle.
(c) only when the fusimotor fibres supplying the spindle are stimulated.
(d) in the presence of extrafusal shortening provided there is sufficient accompanying intrafusal shortening.

7 Golgi tendon organs in skeletal muscle are located:
(a) in the tendon, close to the point of termination of several muscle fibres.
(b) between the muscle fibres, within the belly of the muscle.
(c) in the tendon, close to where the tendon attaches to the bone.
(d) within a muscle fibre, close to where the fibre joins the tendon.

8 Golgi tendon organs:
(a) are silenced when a muscle is stretched.
(b) inhibit the discharge of muscle spindles.
(c) produce inhibition of the motoneurones of their own muscle when they are activated.
(d) behave as receptors in parallel with contracting muscle fibres.

9 Golgi tendon organs are:
(a) stimulated by muscle contraction.
(b) found only in extensor muscles.
(c) found primarily in the visceral (internal) organs.
(d) supplied by the fastest conducting afferent fibres in the body.

10 Activity in a muscle's tendon organs:
(a) results in increased excitability of motoneurones in that muscle.
(b) produces, via a monosynaptic reflex, rapid shortening of synergist muscles.
(c) elicits a crossed flexor reflex.
(d) results in increased excitability of antagonist motoneurones.

11 In non-hairy or glabrous skin:
(a) the absence of hair basket endings results in a reduced range of somatic sensibility.
(b) there is an excess of free-branching nerve endings compared with hairy skin.
(c) Meissner corpuscles are common.
(d) there are no rapidly adapting mechanoreceptors.

12 A dendrite of a nerve cell:
(a) is a low threshold region and the site of initiation of the action potential.
(b) receives the synaptic terminals of other nerve cells.
(c) consists of the presynaptic arborization and nerve terminals of that cell.
(d) is a myelinated axonal extension terminating at a sensory receptor.

13 Excitatory postsynaptic potentials (EPSPs) are:
(a) not produced by any chemical transmitter.
(b) capable of temporal and spatial summation.
(c) not produced by an increase in the permeability of the postsynaptic membrane to positively charged ions.
(d) produced by a specific increase in the permeability of the postsynaptic membrane to chloride ions.

14 Excitatory postsynaptic potentials:
(a) spread passively up to the initial segment region of the motoneurone before they are likely to trigger an action potential.
(b) are generated as the result of a non-specific increase in permeability to small anions.
(c) are a necessary accompaniment of presynaptic inhibition.
(d) can be distinguished from the endplate potentials at the neuromuscular junction by the fact that single endplate potentials are never large enough to trigger an action potential in the muscle fibre.

15 Excitatory synaptic action is:
(a) not influenced by any pharmacological agents.
(b) capable of temporal and spatial summation.
(c) an all-or-nothing response.
(d) of shorter duration than an action potential.

16 Which statement about the excitatory synaptic potentials recorded from a motoneurone following stimulation of the appropriate afferent nerve is INCORRECT?
(a) Their time course is mainly dictated by the passive electrical properties of the neurone.
(b) They are due to the release of acetylcholine by the presynaptic terminals.
(c) They are caused by an increase in conductance for cations.
(d) They are graded as opposed to all-or-nothing events.

17 Excitatory synaptic potentials can be distinguished from inhibitory synaptic potentials. Which statement is CORRECT? Excitatory synaptic potentials:
(a) result only from an increase in membrane permeability while inhibitory synaptic potentials result only from a decrease in membrane permeability.
(b) result only from a decrease in membrane permeability while inhibitory synaptic potentials result only from an increase in membrane permeability.
(c) always represent membrane depolarization while inhibitory synaptic potential always represent hyperpolarization.
(d) always make a neurone more likely to generate an action potential while inhibitory synaptic potentials make a neurone less likely to generate an action potential.

18 Inhibitory postsynaptic potentials:
(a) unlike excitatory postsynaptic potentials are not conducted passively across the postsynaptic membrane.
(b) are initiated across those portions of postsynaptic membrane which are devoid of synaptic contacts.
(c) are generated by subthreshold depolarization of the presynaptic terminal.
(d) may not always accompany the conductance change triggered by the inhibitory transmitter.

36   Multiple Choice Questions in Physiology

19   Inhibitory transmitters in the spinal cord:
(a) cause a selective increase in conductance for K^+.
(b) cause a decrease in conductance for Na^+.
(c) cause an increase in conductance for Cl^-.
(d) are closely related chemically to glutamate.

20   The receptor potential:
(a) is an all-or-none response of a receptor cell, once threshold has been reached.
(b) results from a specific increase in permeability to K^+.
(c) is a depolarization of the receptor membrane and the amplitude of the depolarization depends on the intensity of the stimulus.
(d) increases gradually in amplitude throughout the period of application of a stimulus of constant intensity.

21   Synaptic potentials are:
(a) recorded in the synaptic cleft and at no other site.
(b) potential changes of the postsynaptic cell produced after the arrival of impulses in presynaptic fibres.
(c) potentials in presynaptic fibres produced by impulses generated in postsynaptic cells.
(d) only inhibitory.

22   Which statement is INCORRECT?
(a) Subthreshold generator potentials set up by two or more appropriate stimuli applied successively to a receptor organ can summate.
(b) Generator potentials are set up by stimulus-evoked changes in membrane ionic conductance.
(c) Generator potentials are abolished by tetrodotoxin.
(d) Generator potentials extend locally and decrementally along the terminals of the afferent fibres.

23   Generator potentials (GP) and synaptic potentials (SP) have many similarities, some of which are listed. Choose the INCORRECT statement. GPs and SPs:
(a) spread passively with decrement from their point of initiation.
(b) have stereotyped amplitudes which cannot be changed.
(c) result from a change in the ionic permeability at the site of initiation.
(d) can still be recorded after voltage-dependent sodium channels have been inactivated.

24 **What region of a nerve cell has the lowest threshold for the generation of an action potential?**
(a) The dendrites.
(b) The axon hillock.
(c) The cell body.
(d) The terminal arborization.

25 **Suppose the membrane potential of a neurone was clamped at the equilibrium potential (Nernst potential) for Cl^-. When a neurotransmitter (NT) is applied to the neurone no current flows across the membrane. Which statement about this experiment is clearly INCORRECT?**
(a) The NT caused an increase in conductance for Cl^-.
(b) The reversal potential for the action of the NT was equal to the Cl^- equilibrium potential.
(c) The NT had an excitatory action since the equilibrium potential for Cl^- is more negative than the resting membrane potential.
(d) It was possible that the NT was that which causes inhibitory synaptic potentials in motoneurones.

26 **A rapidly adapting receptor:**
(a) discharges only (or mainly) at the onset of a steady stimulus.
(b) maintains a high rate of discharge throughout the application of a steady stimulus.
(c) only provides information about the duration of a stimulus.
(d) exhibits a steady generator potential during the application of a steady stimulus.

27 **The threshold stimulus for a receptor is one which:**
(a) is just sufficient to excite the receptor at every trial.
(b) will excite the receptor for 50% of the trials.
(c) just fails to excite the receptor at any trial.
(d) will excite the receptor for 10% of the trials.

28 **An 'adequate' stimulus:**
(a) is that to which a receptor is particularly sensitive.
(b) may cause a rapidly adapting receptor to maintain a high rate of discharge.
(c) is of sufficient intensity that it elicits a response from a receptor of an inappropriate modality.
(d) causes a receptor to respond to 50% of trials.

29 Variations in the intensity of a stimulus affecting a population of receptors:
(a) are signalled partly by the number of sensory units made active by the stimulus.
(b) can only be signalled by changes in firing frequency of sensory fibres.
(c) can be felt only in discrete steps.
(d) are signalled by the strength of the nerve impulses set up by the stimulated sense organs.

30 Information concerning the modality of a stimulus applied to the skin surface:
(a) is largely determined by the number of receptors excited.
(b) is partly supplied by where the fibres of that modality are located in the ascending tracts.
(c) will be determined by the way the generator potentials in each peripheral branch of the axon summate and lead to initiation of an impulse train.
(d) depends on the fact that many receptors of the same type lie alongside one another and have overlapping receptive fields.

31 Which statement is INCORRECT?
(a) Intrafusal muscle fibres are smaller than extrafusal fibres.
(b) Tendon organs are commonly located in the belly of the muscle.
(c) Gamma motoneurones do not innervate extrafusal muscle fibres.
(d) The primary endings of muscle spindles terminate on more than one intrafusal fibre.

32 Fusimotor neurones:
(a) innervate Golgi tendon organs.
(b) have monosynaptic connections with Ia afferent fibres.
(c) provide the efferent innervation of muscle spindles.
(d) have axons that run in the synaptic chain.

33 Which statement is INCORRECT? Increased activity of fusimotor neurones (γ-motoneurones):
(a) alters the sensitivity of Golgi tendon organs.
(b) leads to contraction of intrafusal muscle fibres.
(c) increases the sensitivity of muscle spindles.
(d) produces no direct effect on extrafusal muscle fibres.

34 **The location of the site of sensory stimulation in the periphery is conveyed to the central nervous system:**
(a) exclusively by mechanoreceptors.
(b) by the amplitude of the receptor's generator potential.
(c) by the number of receptors activated.
(d) by the particular group of receptors activated; the location of their fibres within the afferent pathways in the central nervous system.

35 **Interneurones:**
(a) are important in the reflex coordination of muscle action.
(b) exert only excitatory action upon other neurones.
(c) are essential for the stretch (myotatic) reflex.
(d) are found only in the spinal cord.

36 **Which one of the following nerve fibre types is unmyelinated?**
(a) Warm.
(b) Touch.
(c) γ Efferent.
(d) Preganglionic sympathetic.

37 **The motoneurones which innervate skeletal muscles:**
(a) are found in the dorsal regions of the spinal cord.
(b) can give rise to both myelinated and unmyelinated axons.
(c) have axons whose collaterals synapse with Renshaw cells.
(d) receive only excitatory synapses.

38 **In a mammalian motoneurone the action potential occurs first:**
(a) in the dendrites.
(b) in the initial segment.
(c) at any point on the cell soma.
(d) in the presynaptic terminals.

39 **Group I afferent nerve fibres:**
(a) have a high threshold to electrical stimulation.
(b) convey information from skin receptors.
(c) are the fastest-conducting afferent nerve fibres.
(d) are unmyelinated.

40 **Section of a nerve supplying a region of skin:**
(a) results in the loss only of temperature and pain sensation.
(b) produces a weak paralysis as a result of a weakened flexor reflex.
(c) produces a loss of the majority of receptors supplied by large-calibre axons.
(d) blocks the afferent signals from high and low threshold mechanoreceptors equally.

41 'C' fibres:
(a) have a cross-sectional diameter of 2.5 µm.
(b) were observed in a toad sciatic nerve preparation in the practical class by stimulating the nerve with a relatively high voltage and using an oscilloscope sweep speed of 2 ms/division.
(c) may be involved in pain perception in skin and muscle.
(d) have a slow conduction velocity but are usually myelinated.

4 Central neurophysiology

QUESTIONS

1. **Which statement is INCORRECT? Afferent information could be prevented from reaching the spinal cord by:**
   (a) cutting the ventral roots.
   (b) removing the dorsal root ganglia.
   (c) cutting the dorsal roots.
   (d) crushing all peripheral nerves.

2. **A stretch reflex in the cat soleus muscle:**
   (a) also causes the synergistic muscles to contract.
   (b) is maintained by activation of motoneurones by impulses from the motor cortex.
   (c) also causes the antagonistic muscles to contract.
   (d) also produces subliminal excitation of the motoneurones of synergistic muscles.

3. **Which statement about the 'stretch' reflex is INCORRECT?**
   (a) It is possible to evoke this reflex by a brisk but light tap on the tendon of the muscle which is then excited.
   (b) This reflex can be evoked in postural muscles.
   (c) This reflex is most readily evoked in extensor muscles.
   (d) This reflex, in its simplest form, involves a chain of three neurones.

4. **The stretch or myotatic reflex is usually investigated in an animal:**
   (a) which is deeply anaesthetized.
   (b) in which the relevant dorsal roots have been transected.
   (c) which is decerebrate.
   (d) by electrical stimulation of the nerves of synergistic muscles.

5 The tendon jerk:
(a) involves transmission across only one central nervous synapse.
(b) is elicited by rapid shortening of the test muscle.
(c) can only be elicited from flexor muscles.
(d) is a simple means of testing whether afferent input from cutaneous receptors has retained its reflex potency.

6 The flexor reflex is:
(a) mediated by muscle spindles in flexor muscles.
(b) part of the spinal mechanism of locomotion.
(c) not influenced by higher neural centres in the brain.
(d) a complex response to a noxious stimulus.

7 A flexor reflex:
(a) is always accompanied by relaxation of antagonist muscles in the contralateral limb.
(b) is present only after decerebration.
(c) may be produced by noxious stimulation of the skin.
(d) in its simplest form involves only two neurones.

8 There is only one known monosynaptic reflex. The receptors which evoke this reflex are:
(a) Golgi tendon organs.
(b) muscle spindles.
(c) nociceptors.
(d) a combination of Golgi tendon organs and muscle spindles.

9 Ia afferents (muscle spindle afferents) make monosynaptic:
(a) excitatory connections with motoneurones supplying contralateral extensor muscles.
(b) inhibitory connections with motoneurones supplying antagonist muscles.
(c) excitatory connections with specific populations of α-motoneurones.
(d) inhibitory connections with neurones joining the spinocerebellar tract.

10 An adult animal is only capable of making coordinated walking movements:
(a) because of the continuous information about limb position provided by input from muscle spindles and tendon organs.
(b) as a result of the elimination of inappropriate connections during development.
(c) because there is a continuous monitoring of limb position by joint receptors.
(d) provided the spinal cord has been surgically completely isolated from the periphery.

11 Which statement about locomotion is CORRECT?
(a) The mechanism underlying walking is a chain of reflexes.
(b) Information from sensory receptors in the limbs is necessary for walking to take place.
(c) The mechanism underlying walking is a pattern generator within the spinal cord or brain.
(d) If all ventral roots are cut, an animal on a treadmill is still able to walk.

12 Which statement is INCORRECT?
(a) Tendon organ feedback may compensate for muscle fatigue.
(b) Interneurones receiving input from skin and joint may facilitate tendon organ inhibition.
(c) Stretch of the primary endings of muscle spindles of a muscle acting at one joint typically does not have any reflex effects at other joints.
(d) Motor commands originating in the brain do not act directly on the large motoneurones but operate through the muscle spindle loop via the γ-motoneurones.

13 Which statement concerning motoneurones located in the ventral horn of the spinal cord is INCORRECT?
(a) They receive both inhibitory and excitatory synaptic inputs.
(b) They may receive several thousand synaptic inputs.
(c) Some innervate muscle spindles while others innervate extrafusal muscle fibres.
(d) They have collateral branches which provide a powerful synaptic input onto the cell bodies of Ia spindle primary afferent fibres.

14 If injury or disease destroyed the left half of the spinal cord in the upper cervical region in a human being, the resulting symptoms would include:
(a) loss of temperature and pain sensation on the left side of the body.
(b) interference with movement performance in the right leg due to destruction of the corticospinal tract.
(c) lack of awareness of the position of the right arm.
(d) loss of temperature and pain sensation on the right side of the body.

15 Which statement is INCORRECT? Section of the left half of the spinal cord in the thoracic region produces:
(a) interference with movement performance in the left leg due to section of portions of the pyramidal tract.
(b) loss of temperature and pain sensation on the left side of the body.
(c) loss of temperature and pain sensation on the right side of the body.
(d) a lack of precise localization of light touch to the left leg.

16 Many parasympathetic preganglionic neurones lie in the:
(a) cervical region of the spinal cord.
(b) thoracic region of the spinal cord.
(c) sacral region of the spinal cord.
(d) entire spinal cord.

17 The meninges are membranes which:
(a) enclose the brain.
(b) produce cerebrospinal fluid.
(c) insulate neurones from each other.
(d) enclose the superior colliculus.

18 The hypothalamus borders the:
(a) Sylvian aqueduct.
(b) fourth ventricle.
(c) lateral ventricle.
(d) third ventricle.

19 The thalamus is:
(a) the source of nearly all the axons that project to the cerebral cortex.
(b) concerned mainly with vision.
(c) concerned mainly with hearing.
(d) concerned with autonomic regulation.

20 Which one of the following sensations relay to the thalamus via the non-lemniscal (lateral spinothalamic) pathway?
(a) Pain.
(b) Vibration.
(c) Touch.
(d) Proprioception.

21 The dorsal column – medial lemniscal pathway differs from the spinothalamic pathway to the cortex because it:
(a) has a different number of synapses interspersed between the primary afferent fibre and sensory cortex.
(b) is crossed.
(c) transmits information rapidly and precisely.
(d) carries information mainly from nociceptors and thermoreceptors.

22 Pyramidal tract fibres:
(a) arise in the cerebral cortex.
(b) arise in the thalamus.
(c) innervate the cerebellum exclusively.
(d) are concerned in discriminative sensory capacity.

23 The mammalian cerebellum:
(a) receives all its afferent fibres from the retina.
(b) is concerned with the coordination of movement.
(c) receives its afferent input only from proprioceptors in muscle.
(d) is entirely concerned with autonomic regulation.

24 The cerebellum receives input from all the following EXCEPT:
(a) vestibular nuclei.
(b) hypothalamus.
(c) cerebral cortex.
(d) muscle spindles.

25 In the mammalian cerebral cortex:
(a) stimulating the primary motor area produces involuntary contractions of body parts.
(b) information between the left and right hemisphere communicates via the corpus luteum.
(c) all pyramidal cells, by definition, carry information leaving the brain.
(d) the sensory and motor regions lie anatomically widely separated to ensure no unnecessary 'cross-talk'.

26 The mammalian cerebral cortex:
(a) is unaffected by anaesthetics.
(b) demonstrates no activity during sleep.
(c) is necessary for the maintenance of normal rhythmic breathing.
(d) is organized so that different regions subserve different functions.

27 The density of synapses in the cerebral cortex is nearest to:
(a) 10^{20} cm^{-3}.
(b) 10^{12} cm^{-3}.
(c) 10^{4} cm^{-3}.
(d) 10 cm^{-3}.

28 The somatic sensory cortex in humans:
(a) receives axons only from the dorsal column nuclei.
(b) is situated in the pre-central gyrus.
(c) has a representation of body parts proportional in area to their density of innervation.
(d) is necessary for carrying out all postural reflexes.

29 Which statement is CORRECT for an animal in which the arm and the hand regions of the sensory cortex on the right side have been removed?
(a) The left arm will show some deficit in the performance of voluntary movements.
(b) There will be a loss in the left hand of the ability to distinguish between objects by touch.
(c) There will be a loss of pain sensation on both sides of the body.
(d) An interference will occur with temperature sensation on the right side of the body.

30 For an animal which has had the hand region of the motor cortex in the right cerebral hemisphere removed, which statement is CORRECT?
(a) There will be a lack of precise localization of light touch on the left side of the body.
(b) The right hand will show a deficit in the performance of fine manipulations.
(c) There will be a loss of pain sensation on both sides of the body.
(d) The left hand will show a deficit in the performance of voluntary movement.

Central neurophysiology 47

31 The motor cortex of humans:
(a) is situated in the occipital lobe of the cerebrum.
(b) contains neurones which are arranged somatotopically, with the foot being represented medially.
(c) plays a major role in the detection of pain.
(d) projects only to α-motoneurones on the opposite side of the body.

32 The motor cortex of humans:
(a) illustrates somatotopic representation of the body musculature.
(b) is situated in the hind brain.
(c) projects principally to spinal motoneurones on the same side of the body.
(d) is the head ganglion of the sympathetic nervous system.

33 The motor area of the cerebral cortex:
(a) is the site of memory storage.
(b) is the centre commanding the execution of movements.
(c) can be mapped into a number of areas where the different parts of the body are represented equally.
(d) is composed of six different layers, those containing the main outflow being layers 5 and 6.

34 Pyramidal cells in the motor cortex:
(a) all send their axons in the pyramidal tract.
(b) may make monosynaptic connections with interneurones in the spinal cord.
(c) all send their axons to the spinal cord in the corticospinal tract.
(d) receive no sensory input.

35 Which statement is INCORRECT? The EEG:
(a) is a result of activity in thalamocortical neurones.
(b) shows synchronized slow waves during rapid eye movement (paradoxical) sleep.
(c) is measured in microvolts rather than millivolts.
(d) shows desynchronization in response to an unexpected stimulus.

36 Decerebrate rigidity caused by midbrain transection in a cat is:
(a) accompanied by a waking EEG record in the isolated forebrain (*cerveau isolé*).
(b) accompanied by a fixed flexed posture of all four limbs.
(c) increased following damage to the anterior lobe of the cerebellum.
(d) increased following section of all dorsal root afferent fibres.

48 Multiple Choice Questions in Physiology

37 After a period of recovery from the transection, a 'high' decerebrate cat with an intact midbrain:
(a) is unable to right itself if put off balance.
(b) stands with a normal distribution of contraction in extensor and flexor muscles.
(c) is unable to walk on a treadmill.
(d) continuously exhibits exaggerated stretch reflexes in the extensor muscles (decerebrate rigidity).

38 Which statement is INCORRECT?
(a) Sensations of thirst, hunger and cold are triggered in part by signals from peripheral receptors, e.g. in mouth, stomach and skin.
(b) The hypothalamus is involved in regulation of body temperature, drinking and eating.
(c) Stimulation of the labyrinthine organs in the ear (e.g. by motion) may produce nausea and imbalance.
(d) The frontal cortex is essential for coordination of movement.

39 Which statement is INCORRECT?
(a) It is currently thought that the formation of long-term memory involves the synthesis of specific neuronal proteins.
(b) The corpus callosum is essential for the transfer of information from one cerebral hemisphere to the other.
(c) In humans, both cerebral hemispheres are normally involved in the articulation and understanding of speech.
(d) The development of neuronal connections depends upon genetic control and the confirmation of the connections by use.

40 Which statement is INCORRECT?
(a) Damage to precentral (motor) cortex (e.g. by stroke) leads to spastic paralysis on the opposite side of the body.
(b) Colour vision occurs only in bright light which enables the visual cortex to convert by central processing the uniform rod receptor signals into three colour sensations.
(c) Memory formation may be disturbed if the temporal lobe of the brain is damaged.
(d) Electrical signals from cells in one cerebral hemisphere may be carried to the other hemisphere by the corpus callosum.

41 Which statement is INCORRECT?
(a) The pyramidal tract is important for execution of skilled movements.
(b) The main layer of cerebral cortex-containing cells which receives incoming information from the thalamus is layer 4.
(c) Lesions of the cerebellum result in disturbance of posture, gait, muscle tone and motor coordination.
(d) The extrapyramidal pathway includes fibres descending from the cerebral cortex to spinal levels without a synapse.

42 Which statement is INCORRECT?
(a) The afferent pathways of all sensory modalities, with the exception of smell, make synaptic connections within the thalamus.
(b) The dorsal column medial lemniscal pathway exhibits precise somatotopic organization.
(c) Fibres of the spinothalamic tract synapse with neurones in the dorsal horn before crossing to the opposite side of the spinal cord and ascending to the thalamus.
(d) The somatic sensory cortex in humans is situated in the frontal lobe.

43 Which statement is INCORRECT?
(a) Lesions of the cerebellum result in disturbances of posture, gait, muscle tone and motor coordination.
(b) The pyramidal tract is not important in the control of the skilled actions of the distal limb musculature.
(c) The extrapyramidal pathways are a complex system of fibre tracts and nuclei which include the basal ganglia and motor nuclei in the brainstem.
(d) Purkinje neurones are the only output cells of the cerebellum and have an inhibitory action on neurones in the cerebellar nuclei.

44 Which statement is INCORRECT?
(a) Damage to the cerebellum results in the loss of fine motor skills on the opposite side of the body.
(b) Motor areas in the cerebral cortex of primates project some fibres directly to α-motoneurones, but most end on interneurones.
(c) The extrapyramidal motor system is mainly involved in the organization of complex automatic body movements and posture.
(d) Focal electrical stimulation of the motor cortex causes movement in discrete groups of muscles on the opposite side of the body.

45 **Which statement is CORRECT?**
(a) The dorsal columns receive collaterals from all afferent fibres other than from muscle.
(b) In the sensory cortex somatic representation is not proportional to area of skin surface.
(c) Ablation of the anterior lobe of the cerebellum produces muscle weakness on one side of the body.
(d) All of the small freely branching endings in the skin are insensitive to mechanical stimuli and subserve only the sensations of pain or temperature.

5 Sensory physiology

QUESTIONS

1 Which statement is CORRECT?
(a) Taste and smell pathways run together in the brain.
(b) The taste pathway terminates in the same cortical area as other sensory fibres from the tongue.
(c) Olfactory fibres terminate in the 'nose-area' of the somatosensory cortex.
(d) A small discrete group of high molecular weight substances is responsible for the sense of smell.

2 Primary afferent nerve fibres from taste receptors:
(a) each respond specifically to a particular chemical stimulus.
(b) adapt in their firing rate to maintained application of the taste stimulus to the tongue.
(c) proceed to the thalamus without interruption.
(d) represent dendritic processes of bud cells.

3 Taste buds:
(a) are distributed evenly over the tongue.
(b) send their axons to the medial geniculate body.
(c) respond preferentially to different substances.
(d) respond in exactly the same way to different substances, and encode different sensation by virtue of their connection.

4 Which statement is CORRECT?
(a) Olfactory receptor cells release a chemical transmitter on to olfactory nerve terminals.
(b) There are four basic qualities of odour, and the receptors for these are segregated within each nasal mucosa.
(c) Olfactory receptor cell potentials increase in magnitude with increases in concentration of odoriferous substances.
(d) All olfactory nerve fibres are activated by a highly discrete group of substances which differs from fibre to fibre.

5 Which of the following statements is INCORRECT?
(a) Each olfactory receptor cell is activated by a discrete range of substances.
(b) Olfactory cells do not discriminate between different chemical substances.
(c) When damaged, olfactory cells can regenerate.
(d) Olfactory stimuli need to have low molecular weights.

6 With respect to taste:
(a) sweet substances may taste unpleasant at low concentrations.
(b) there is an increase in the number of taste buds up to the age of 45 years.
(c) there are only four flavours which correspond to the four primary tastes.
(d) there is no adaptation in firing rates in taste afferent fibres and all adaptation takes place within the brain.

7 Which statement is CORRECT?
(a) Different taste sensations are entirely due to the separation of taste buds subserving the five basic taste senses on the tongue.
(b) Only one taste nerve fibre supplies each taste bud.
(c) The normal life span of a taste cell is much shorter than that of a cochlear hair cell.
(d) Unlike the olfactory system, there is a simple relationship between chemical structure and taste sensation.

8 Which statement is CORRECT?
(a) All taste nerve fibres are gathered together in one cranial nerve.
(b) Neurones in the medial geniculate nucleus respond to taste stimuli.
(c) The olfactory pathway in the brain exactly parallels that of the visual system.
(d) No thalamic nucleus subserving olfaction is present.

Sensory physiology 53

9 Which statement concerning substances which produce olfactory sensitivities is INCORRECT? They are:
(a) volatile substances.
(b) substances which are gases at body temperature.
(c) water-soluble substances.
(d) lipid-soluble substances.

10 Which statement is CORRECT? Taste:
(a) receptor cells are depolarized only by one type of substance.
(b) nerve fibres discharge maximally in response to one type of substance.
(c) information is not transmitted to the sensory cortex.
(d) cells, like hair cells, are irreplaceable in the adult.

11 Olfactory receptor cells:
(a) are distributed uniformly throughout the nasal cavity.
(b) regenerate within 24 hours after damage.
(c) are specialized neurones.
(d) release a chemical transmitter on to olfactory nerve terminals.

12 To which substance are our taste receptors most sensitive (on a molar basis)?
(a) Sucrose.
(b) Sodium chloride.
(c) Quinine.
(d) Strychnine.

13 Olfactory receptors:
(a) occur in all parts of the nose except the nasal mucosa.
(b) in large numbers are connected to each individual olfactory nerve fibres.
(c) are each responsive only to a unique substance.
(d) are not represented in the sensory neocortex.

14 Individual taste buds:
(a) can be classed into one of four types according to the number of receptor cells and the pattern of innervation.
(b) detect only one of the four principal tastes, and are unresponsive to the other three.
(c) are innervated by one afferent fibre.
(d) tend to show a preferential sensitivity to one of the four principal tastes.

15 Semicircular canals:
(a) are stimulated during changes in angular velocity of head movement.
(b) are insensitive to changes in angular velocity but relay information only during steady movements of the head in one direction.
(c) are receptors for air pressure.
(d) when stimulated, produce optokinetic nystagmus.

16 Which statement is INCORRECT?
(a) Pressure is amplified in the middle ear because of an area difference between eardrum and oval window.
(b) The middle ear muscles contract due to both acoustic and non-acoustic influences.
(c) Drainage of fluid from the middle ear will lead to a hearing loss.
(d) The lever ratio of the middle ear ossicular chain is approximately 1.3.

17 Which statement is INCORRECT?
(a) Synapses from cochlear nerve fibres are located at the bases of hair cells.
(b) Hair cells release a chemical transmitter onto cochlear nerve terminals.
(c) Hair cells are specialized dendrites of cochlear neurones.
(d) The interior of a hair cell is at a more negative potential than endolymph.

18 The basilar membrane, when stimulated:
(a) vibrates maximally at the apex to high sound frequency.
(b) behaves as though uniformly elastic from base to apex.
(c) will not respond at the base to low frequencies.
(d) behaves as though a travelling wave passes along it.

19 The brain auditory pathway:
(a) has relays in the cochlear nucleus, medial geniculate body and auditory cortex.
(b) is entirely uncrossed.
(c) differs from the visual and somatosensory systems in showing no topographic organization.
(d) does not utilize the time pattern of impulses in its coding mechanism.

20 A low-frequency sound:
(a) can excite most auditory nerve fibres provided it is intense enough.
(b) is coded for only by the outer row of hair cells.
(c) can be signalled by all auditory neurones, provided it is 10 000 Hz or more.
(d) will be signalled only by hair cells lying on the basal segment of basilar membrane.

21 Which statement about the external ear is INCORRECT?
(a) The pinna is considered to be part of the external ear.
(b) The external auditory canal is considered to be part of the external ear.
(c) The stapedius muscle is considered to be part of the external ear.
(d) The external ear behaves like an organ pipe tuned to the sound frequencies best heard by the listener.

22 Which one of the following is NOT concerned with the reflexes associated with rotational stimuli?
(a) Tectorial membrane.
(b) Cupula.
(c) Vestibular nerve.
(d) Endolymph.

23 Hair cells in the horizontal vestibular semicircular canal system:
(a) are modified dendrites of axons from the vestibular nuclei.
(b) are depolarized by cupula movements away from the utricle.
(c) contain perilymph.
(d) release a chemical transmitter on to afferent nerve terminals.

24 A sound of 0 decibels SPL (sound pressure level) has a pressure:
(a) one-tenth of that of the threshold pressure.
(b) ten times that of the threshold pressure.
(c) equal to zero.
(d) equal to the threshold pressure.

25 The afferent transmitter between hair cells and cochlear nerve endings is:
(a) acetylcholine.
(b) noradrenaline.
(c) dopamine.
(d) none of the above.

26 Perilymph:
(a) has a high concentration of potassium ions.
(b) is secreted by the hair cells.
(c) is equipotential with extracellular fluid.
(d) fills the semicircular canals.

27 The middle ear structures serve to amplify the sound pressure initially registered at the eardrum mainly because the:
(a) ligaments connecting the bones are unusually flexible.
(b) tympanic membrane is approximately 20 times larger in area than the oval window.
(c) air pressure within the middle ear cavity is one-third of that outside.
(d) external auditory meatus has a characteristic resonant frequency.

28 Constant loud noise may cause a high-frequency hearing loss because:
(a) all vibrations pass through the base of the cochlea.
(b) hair cells responding to high frequencies are very fragile.
(c) middle ear ossicles are easily dislocated by high frequencies.
(d) loud noise damages nerve fibres in the ear.

29 One after-effect of a long period of rotation to the right is:
(a) rapid (saccadic) components of eye movements directed to the right.
(b) slow components of eye movements to the right.
(c) past pointing to the left.
(d) none of the above.

30 Which statement is CORRECT?
(a) The basilar membrane vibrates in a standing wave pattern.
(b) Perilymph is found in both the cochlea and the semicircular canals.
(c) The most sensitively heard frequency is identical to the dominant frequency in human adult speech.
(d) The majority of cochlear nerve fibres originate from the inner hair cells.

31 Inner hair cells:
(a) are the dendrites of cochlear nerve fibres.
(b) contain endolymph.
(c) are more common than outer hair cells.
(d) cannot regenerate in the adult.

32 Endolymph:
(a) occurs in scala vestibuli.
(b) occurs in scala media.
(c) is rich in sodium ions.
(d) is rich in chloride ions.

33 Nerve impulses in the auditory nerve convey information about the pitch of a high-frequency sound:
(a) according to the average frequency of impulses in all axons.
(b) by a particular axon being active while all the rest are inactive.
(c) by all the axons firing in time with the sound wave.
(d) according to which axons are active.

34 At the commencement of rotation of a blindfolded subject in a chair his or her:
(a) eye movements are dependent on visual input.
(b) eyes flick in the direction of rotation and then drift in the opposite direction.
(c) eye movements stop.
(d) eyes drift in the direction of rotation and then flick in the opposite direction.

35 Endolymph:
(a) has a high concentration of sodium ions.
(b) has a positive charge compared with perilymph.
(c) is secreted by hair cells.
(d) is equipotential with extracellular fluid.

36 The basilar membrane:
(a) has uniform mechanical properties from base to apex.
(b) vibrates at most points to low frequencies.
(c) only responds at the base to low frequencies.
(d) vibrates with a standing wave pattern to all frequencies.

37 The chief refracting surface in the human eye is the:
(a) retina.
(b) posterior surface of the lens.
(c) anterior corneal surface.
(d) anterior surface of the lens.

38 Which statement is INCORRECT?
(a) Ganglion cells in the mammalian retina discharge in the dark.
(b) Ganglion cells in the peripheral retina are insensitive to low levels of illumination and only respond in daylight.
(c) Retinene is synthesized from vitamin A stored in the pigmented epithelium.
(d) Glaucoma is caused by an excessive elevation in the intraocular pressure.

39 Which statement is CORRECT?
(a) A person with deuteranopia cannot see red.
(b) A rod monochromat can only recognize blue.
(c) The ability to recognize yellow-green hues depends on the retinal pigment rhodopsin.
(d) A person with protanopia might be unable to tell a red tie from a black tie.

40 Section of the human optic tract on one side produces:
(a) total blindness in one eye.
(b) a loss of sensation to light rays falling on both the contralateral nasal retina and ipsilateral temporal retina.
(c) a loss of sensation to light rays falling on both the ipsilateral nasal retina and contralateral temporal retina.
(d) a disturbance of binocular vision for objects in the entire visual world.

41 The primary visual pathways in the brain:
(a) are entirely crossed.
(b) carry information only about the left eye on the left side of the brain.
(c) carry information mainly about the right visual field on the left side of the brain.
(d) include direct connections from one retina to the other.

42 Cones:
(a) always use rhodopsin as photopigment but have specialized interconnections with bipolar cells.
(b) only occur at the fovea.
(c) are hyperpolarized by light.
(d) function best at very low light intensities.

43 Presbyopia is most common in:
(a) men.
(b) women.
(c) old people.
(d) young people.

44 At the human fovea, the high visual acuity is due to a concentration of:
(a) blood vessels nourishing the receptors.
(b) low-light threshold rod receptors.
(c) higher-threshold cone receptors.
(d) optic nerve fibres.

45 When refractive power differs in different meridians of the eye, the person is:
(a) myopic.
(b) hypermetropic.
(c) presbyopic.
(d) astigmatic.

46 An object which is 1 cm in diameter placed 1 m from a subject with a reduced eye equal to 2 cm will focus to a spot on the retina with a diameter of about:
(a) 2 μm.
(b) 200 μm.
(c) 2 mm.
(d) 200 mm.

47 The thalamic nucleus receiving optic nerve fibres is the:
(a) medial geniculate nucleus.
(b) ventrobasal complex.
(c) lateral geniculate nucleus.
(d) visual cortex.

48 During visual accommodation the ciliary muscles:
(a) relax, thus releasing tension from the zonular fibres.
(b) contract but the iris relaxes.
(c) and the iris contract.
(d) contract, increasing tension on the zonular fibres.

49 Retinal photoreceptors:
(a) are inactive in the dark.
(b) are depolarized by light.
(c) are hyperpolarized by light.
(d) all contain rhodopsin.

50 **Which statement is CORRECT?**
(a) The cornea may be transplanted because it has no nerve supply.
(b) The iris muscle is supplied with both sympathetic and parasympathetic nerve fibres.
(c) The ciliary muscle only receives sympathetic innervation.
(d) The vitreous humour separates the lens and cornea.

51 **The optic surface in the human eye producing greatest refraction is the:**
(a) anterior corneal surface.
(b) posterior corneal surface.
(c) anterior surface of the lens.
(d) posterior surface of the lens.

52 **Light shone into one eye of a dark-adapted subject would be expected to result in nerve fibres of the:**
(a) parasympathetic system causing the opposite pupil to constrict.
(b) sympathetic system causing the opposite pupil to dilate.
(c) sympathetic system causing the pupil to constrict.
(d) parasympathetic system causing the pupil to dilate.

53 **Points on the left side of the visual field are represented on the:**
(a) nasal side of the retinae.
(b) right side of the retinae.
(c) lateral side of the retinae.
(d) left side of the retinae.

54 **The retina:**
(a) is structured so that photoreceptors receive light reflected off the chorioid.
(b) utilizes a single photopigment which has different effects on rod and cone function.
(c) contains receptor cells whose axons comprise the optic nerve.
(d) is active in the dark.

55 **The fovea is the:**
(a) tissue attached to the ciliary muscle.
(b) retinal region of entry and exit of blood vessels and optic nerve fibres.
(c) region of retina which intersects with the visual axis of the eye.
(d) blind spot.

Sensory physiology

56 Which one of the following is the most direct pathway for visual information travelling from the retina to the visual cortex?
(a) retina→superior colliculus→inferior olive→visual cortex
(b) retina→optic tract →lateral geniculate→visual cortex
(c) retina→oculomotor nucleus→visual cortex
(d) retina→lateral geniculate→superior colliculus→visual cortex

57 Sensory pathways in the central nervous system:
(a) except for the auditory system, are topographically organized.
(b) include primary afferent nerve fibres whose discharges adapt with maintained stimulation.
(c) are identical in terms of the number of synaptic interruptions and differ only in terms of the receptors which activate them.
(d) represent the receptor sheet equally, irrespective of peripheral innervation density.

58 In the mammalian special sense organs, single nerve fibres:
(a) in the olfactory mucosa show rapid adaptation to a repeated olfactory stimulus.
(b) in the auditory nerve show larger action potentials in response to louder sounds.
(c) in the innervation of the semicircular canals are insensitive to thermal convection currents in the canals.
(d) innervating taste buds often respond to more than one taste substance.

59 Central pathways for hearing, vision and somatic sensation:
(a) have identical connections and differ only in their receptor mechanisms.
(b) utilize varied patterns of central connection but have the same receptor mechanisms.
(c) all terminate in specific sensory cortical areas.
(d) show no topographic organization beyond the thalamus.

60 Each individual nerve fibre:
(a) in the optic nerve will respond when light falls on any part of the retina.
(b) in the auditory nerve has larger action potentials in response to louder sounds.
(c) originating from the semicircular canals is insensitive to thermal convection currents in the canals.
(d) originating from taste buds adapts in its firing rate when a chemical substance remains in contact with the taste bud.

61 Which statement is INCORRECT?
(a) Gross sensory qualities (vision, hearing, etc.) arise by virtue of WHICH brain pathway is stimulated, not HOW it is stimulated.
(b) All sensory pathways include a separate, non-neural receptor cell.
(c) The first, second and eighth cranial nerves are sensory nerves.
(d) Topographic organization concerns the way different receptor surfaces are mapped on to populations of neurones in the brain.

62 The cornea may be transplanted because it:
(a) receives oxygen from air and fluids.
(b) is a gel-like matrix of protein.
(c) has no nerve supply.
(d) does not require oxygen for its survival.

63 During accommodation of the eye to near points the:
(a) posterior surface of the lens bulges forward.
(b) ciliary muscle relaxes, allowing the lens to change shape.
(c) ciliary and circular iris muscles contract.
(d) eye becomes suited to far vision.

64 Which statement is CORRECT?
(a) Each cone is responsive to only one wavelength of light.
(b) Cone photopigments are differently coloured retinene.
(c) Colour blindness is more common among females than males.
(d) Rods may respond to lights of different wavelengths.

65 Which statement is INCORRECT?
(a) The activities of many rods converge on to a single ganglion cell in the peripheral retina.
(b) Form vision is a property of foveal cone systems.
(c) Movement detection is a property of peripheral rod systems.
(d) Colour detection cannot occur outside the fovea.

6 Autonomic nervous system

QUESTIONS

1 Synaptic transmission is considered to be chemically mediated because:
(a) it can occur in both directions at a synapse.
(b) there is no delay in transmission across the synapse.
(c) presynaptic and postsynaptic potential changes have the same time-course.
(d) it can be influenced by drugs which affect chemical agents presumed to be transmitters.

2 Which statement about the autonomic nervous system is CORRECT?
(a) Transmission velocity in postganglionic autonomic nerves is about the same as that in somatic motor nerves.
(b) The ratio of the number of preganglionic : postganglionic fibres is about 20 : 1.
(c) Sympathetic vasoconstrictor nerves supply the smooth muscle in the walls of arterioles almost everywhere in the body.
(d) There are also parasympathetic vasodilator nerves that supply arterioles in striated muscles.

3 Which statement is INCORRECT?
(a) Parasympathetic postganglionic neurones occur very close to the tissues they innervate.
(b) Acetylcholine is the transmitter at all ganglionic synapses and at all sympathetic neuroeffector junctions.
(c) Sympathetic postganglionic neurones occur at a distance from the tissues they innervate.
(d) All efferent fibres leaving the spinal cord of the somatic and autonomic nervous system release acetylcholine which acts on nicotinic receptors.

4 Which one of the following does the vagus nerve NOT innervate?
(a) Heart.
(b) Parotid gland.
(c) Oesophagus.
(d) Small intestine.

5 Which one of the following is NOT caused by stimulation of the vagus?
(a) Slowing of the heart.
(b) Constriction of the lower oesophageal sphincter.
(c) Constriction of the bronchioles.
(d) Increased motility of the small intestine.

6 Stimulation of the vagus leads to:
(a) constriction of the pupil.
(b) increase in mobility of the gastrointestinal tract.
(c) increased cardiac contractility.
(d) relaxation of the bronchioles.

7 An example of a paravertebral ganglion is the:
(a) stellate ganglion.
(b) coeliac ganglion.
(c) superior mesenteric ganglion.
(d) inferior mesenteric ganglion.

8 Which statement regarding autonomic preganglionic fibres is INCORRECT? Preganglionic:
(a) fibres are myelinated B fibres.
(b) nerve cell bodies lie in the central nervous system.
(c) fibres can directly innervate effector organs.
(d) fibres are only excitatory.

9 Which statement is INCORRECT?
(a) Preganglionic fibres are non-myelinated B fibres.
(b) Postganglionic fibres are non-myelinated C fibres.
(c) Lower motor neurone fibres are usually myelinated A fibres.
(d) Motor fibres leaving the central nervous system usually release acetylcholine.

10 Ganglion-blocking drugs were used primarily to:
(a) depress the rate of heart beat.
(b) increase gastric acid secretion.
(c) prevent convulsions in strychnine poisoning.
(d) combat hypertension.

11 Ganglion-blocking drugs are much less frequently used at present because they:
(a) cause parasympathetic blockade.
(b) block muscarinic receptors.
(c) block all nicotinic receptors throughout the body.
(d) block α-receptors.

12 Which one of the following is NOT characteristic of the sympathetic nervous system?
(a) Extensive branching of individual axons.
(b) Multiple synaptic inputs.
(c) No tonic activity.
(d) Filtering of information.

13 Which one of the following does NOT result from stimulation of the sympathetic nervous system?
(a) Increased sweating.
(b) A 'goose' flesh.
(c) Increased gastrointestinal motility.
(d) Pupillary dilatation.

14 The sympathetic nervous system may be distinguished from the parasympathetic system because:
(a) the transmitter at preganglionic terminals in sympathetic ganglia can be noradrenaline but is always acetylcholine in parasympathetic ganglia.
(b) sympathetic ganglia have only nicotinic receptors, while parasympathetic ganglia have only muscarinic receptors.
(c) the transmitter at the postganglionic sympathetic terminals is always noradrenaline, while at the parasympathetic postganglionic terminals, the transmitter is always acetylcholine.
(d) the sympathetic system causes inhibition in the gastrointestinal tract, while the parasympathetic is excitatory.

15 Which one of the following cranial nerves does NOT contain parasympathetic fibres?
(a) Optic nerve (II).
(b) Facial nerve (VII).
(c) Glossopharyngeal nerve (IX).
(d) Vagus nerve (X).

16 Many parasympathetic preganglionic neurones lie in the:
(a) cervical region of the spinal cord.
(b) thoracic region of the spinal cord.
(c) sacral region of the spinal cord.
(d) entire spinal cord.

17 Which one of the following cranial nerves contains parasympathetic fibres?
(a) Facial.
(b) Hypoglossal.
(c) Optic.
(d) Vestibulo-cochlear.

18 Which one of the following is NOT caused by activation of parasympathetic nerve fibres?
(a) Defaecation.
(b) Micturition.
(c) Erection.
(d) Ejaculation of semen.

19 Which one of the following is NOT caused by stimulation of the parasympathetic system?
(a) Lacrimation.
(b) Increased gastrointestinal motility.
(c) Engorgement of genital erectile tissue.
(d) Increased cardiac contractility.

20 A partial agonist:
(a) will, in sufficient quantities, produce a response as large as a true agonist.
(b) will never reduce the effect of a true agonist if both drugs are present simultaneously.
(c) has a dose–response curve that is flatter than that of a true agonist.
(d) always has a lower affinity for the receptor than a true agonist.

21 Which statement concerning agonist and antagonist drug action on a receptor is INCORRECT?
(a) An antagonist may have a higher affinity than an agonist for a receptor.
(b) Antagonists have no efficacy.
(c) Different agonists may have similar potencies but have different efficacies.
(d) Different agonists with similar efficacy have similar affinity for a receptor.

Autonomic nervous system

22 A purely competitive antagonist:
(a) depresses the maximum response of a tissue to an applied agonist.
(b) shifts the log-dose–response curve for an agonist to the right.
(c) can itself activate receptors.
(d) can cause a change in the slope of the agonist log-dose–response curve.

23 Competitive antagonists:
(a) always depress the response that a tissue produces whatever the concentration of agonist.
(b) always cause the slope of the log-dose–response agonist curve to be changed.
(c) always cause a parallel shift of the log-dose–response curve.
(d) in any concentration never occupy most of the receptors in a tissue.

24 A non-competitive antagonist:
(a) in any concentration always depresses the maximum response of a tissue to an applied agonist.
(b) cannot be washed from a tissue after a long exposure to the tissue.
(c) may cause a change in the slope of the relationship between agonist concentration and response.
(d) can itself activate receptors.

25 An intravenous injection of adrenaline into an anaesthetized cat would:
(a) accelerate the heart rate.
(b) greatly increase gastric acid secretion.
(c) constrict the pupil.
(d) cause a prolonged increase of salivary secretion.

26 The adrenal medulla secretes adrenaline in response to administration of:
(a) atropine.
(b) tubocurarine.
(c) methyldopa.
(d) nicotine.

27 Noradrenaline:
(a) only activates α-receptors.
(b) is the only catecholamine present in mammals.
(c) only activates β-receptors.
(d) is mainly inactivated by uptake into adrenergic nerve terminals.

28 Inhibition of noradrenaline uptake by sympathetic postganglionic axons:
(a) produces no change in the apparent sensitivity of the appropriate organ to noradrenaline.
(b) very rapidly leads to a depletion of noradrenaline in those nerves.
(c) causes an increased concentration of noradrenaline metabolites in the urine.
(d) results from an infusion of atropine.

29 Which one of the following does NOT inhibit noradrenaline release?
(a) Guanethidine.
(b) Bretylium.
(c) Bethanidine.
(d) Practolol.

30 In the normal synthetic pathway for noradrenaline:
(a) synthesis of dopamine precedes the synthesis of dihydroxyphenylalanine.
(b) synthesis of adrenaline precedes the synthesis of noradrenaline.
(c) dihydroxyphenylalanine is converted directly to noradrenaline.
(d) dopamine β-hydroxylase catalyses the synthesis of noradrenaline from dopamine.

31 Which one of the following drugs does NOT affect synthesis of noradrenaline?
(a) Phentolamine.
(b) α-Methyldopa.
(c) α-Methyl p-tyrosine.
(d) 6-Hydroxydopamine.

32 Addition of noradrenaline to the medium surrounding an isolated mammalian heart preparation causes:
(a) no effect, because it acts only on α-receptors.
(b) an acceleration because it has strong α-stimulating properties.
(c) a slowing of the heart, because it stimulates vagal nerve endings.
(d) an acceleration, because it acts on cardiac β-receptors.

33 When noradrenaline is injected into an intact anaesthetized animal it results in:
(a) increase in both heart rate and blood pressure.
(b) inhibition of the intestinal motility.
(c) decrease in both heart rate and blood pressure.
(d) constriction of the pupil.

Autonomic nervous system

34 Noradrenaline, when applied to an isolated frog or toad heart, causes an increase in the rate of beating. The potency of noradrenaline on this isolated organ would be augmented by pretreatment with:
(a) cocaine.
(b) curare.
(c) propranolol.
(d) atropine.

35 Stimulation of the sympathetic outflow ultimately causes pupillary dilatation because noradrenaline:
(a) contracts radial pupillary muscle.
(b) inhibits the contraction of radial pupillary muscle.
(c) constricts the constrictor pupillary muscle.
(d) inhibits the constriction of constrictor pupillary muscle.

36 Which one of the following statements does NOT distinguish between the two types of receptors to catecholamines (α and β)?
(a) α-Receptors can be blocked by phentolamine whereas β-receptors can be blocked by propranolol.
(b) α-Receptors and β-receptors can be activated by noradrenaline whereas only β-receptors can be activated by isoprenaline.
(c) Activation of α-receptors leads directly to an increase in ion permeability of the cell membrane whereas activation of β-receptors leads initially to a changed biochemical status.
(d) Arterioles possess mainly α-receptors whereas the heart possesses mainly β-receptors.

37 Which statement is INCORRECT?
(a) The smooth muscle of the respiratory tract has a predominance of β_1-receptors.
(b) The smooth muscle in blood vessels has α- and β_2-receptors.
(c) The heart (cardiac muscle) has predominantly β_1-receptors.
(d) The uterus has α- and β_2-receptors.

38 Which one of the following does not contain β_2-receptors?
(a) Uterine smooth muscle.
(b) Blood vessels.
(c) Cardiac muscle.
(d) Respiratory tract smooth muscle.

39 Which one of the following is a specific α_2 agonist?
(a) Isoprenaline.
(b) Tyramine.
(c) Salbutamol.
(d) Metaraminol.

40 Which one of the following drugs is a β-receptor antagonist?
(a) Propranolol.
(b) Phentolamine.
(c) Phenoxybenzamine.
(d) Piperoxan.

41 If an animal was pre-treated with an irreversible α-blocking drug such as phenoxybenzamine, and was then given an intravenous injection of $1\,\mu g\,kg^{-1}$ of adrenaline, which one of the following events would occur?
(a) Vasoconstriction.
(b) Vasodilatation.
(c) Slowing of the heart.
(d) A marked increase in gastric secretion.

42 The drug guanethidine lowers the blood pressure because it:
(a) blocks β-receptors.
(b) prevents noradrenaline synthesis.
(c) blocks α-receptors.
(d) prevents the release of noradrenaline from sympathetic nerves.

43 Guanethidine, an adrenergic neurone blocking agent:
(a) produces blockade of all sympathetic reflexes.
(b) prevents synaptic transmission at sympathetic ganglia.
(c) produces no decrease in sensitivity to externally applied noradrenaline.
(d) facilitates the inactivation of noradrenaline.

44 If a person who had been taking therapeutic doses of guanethidine for several weeks was to rise suddenly to his or her feet from a recumbent position, which one of the following reactions would be most likely to occur in heart rate (HR) and in blood pressure (BP) measured at the brachial artery?
(a) HR increased, BP unchanged.
(b) HR increased, BP decreased.
(c) HR little changed, BP decreased.
(d) HR decreased, BP decreased.

Autonomic nervous system

45 During transmission through autonomic ganglia, acetylcholine activates:
(a) muscarinic receptors and causes an increase in potassium permeability.
(b) nicotinic receptors and causes an increase in sodium permeability alone.
(c) muscarinic receptors and causes an increase in permeability to all cations.
(d) nicotinic receptors and causes an increase in permeability to all cations.

46 Which statement is INCORRECT?
(a) Acetylcholinesterase is important for inactivation of acetylcholine.
(b) Acetylcholinesterase can be inhibited by cimetidine.
(c) Acetylcholinesterase has an anionic and esteratic site for combination with acetylcholine.
(d) There are several different types of cholinesterase.

47 Nicotinic receptors:
(a) always mediate relaxation in smooth muscle.
(b) are stimulated by low doses of acetyl β-methylcholine.
(c) can be blocked by low doses of atropine.
(d) are important in neuromuscular transmission.

48 Which one of the following drugs is NOT a cholinomimetic substance at nicotinic receptors?
(a) Carbachol.
(b) Tetramethylammonium (TMA).
(c) Dimethylphenylpiperazinium (DMPP).
(d) Methacholine.

49 Which one of the following is NOT cholinomimetic at nicotinic receptors?
(a) Nicotine.
(b) Tetramethylammonium (TMA).
(c) Mecamylamine.
(d) Dimethylphenylpiperazinium (DMPP).

50 Nicotine:
(a) stimulates α-receptors.
(b) directly stimulates cardiac muscle.
(c) depresses acetylcholine release from parasympathetic nerve endings.
(d) stimulates sympathetic ganglia.

51 Prolonged exposure of a ganglion to nicotine eventually produces ganglionic blockade because:
(a) nicotine abolishes the release of transmitter from preganglionic terminals.
(b) the equilibrium potential for Na^+ ions becomes 0 mV.
(c) nicotine inhibits the hydrolysis of transmitter.
(d) prolonged exposure of receptors to an agonist causes them to be unresponsive to agonists.

52 Which one of the following effects would be produced by an injection of a large dose of the alkaloid nicotine into an anaesthetized animal?
(a) A prolonged fall in heart rate.
(b) A prolonged constriction of the pupil.
(c) A prolonged enhancement of ganglionic transmission.
(d) A large output of adrenal catecholamines.

53 Which statement is INCORRECT? Nicotinic and muscarinic receptors:
(a) can be activated by acetylcholine.
(b) when activated always results in an increase in Na^+ permeability in the appropriate effector cell.
(c) have dissimilar distributions.
(d) are sequentially activated by both some sympathetic reflexes and some parasympathetic reflexes.

54 Muscarinic receptors:
(a) are present in most involuntary organs.
(b) can be activated by nicotine.
(c) can only be activated by muscarine.
(d) when activated always increase the heart rate.

55 Muscarinic receptors:
(a) always mediate relaxation of smooth muscle.
(b) are important in skeletal neuromuscular transmission.
(c) react primarily to histamine.
(d) can be blocked by low doses of atropine.

56 If a man is treated with a dose of atropine sufficient to block most of his peripheral muscarinic receptors, which one of the following events will occur?
(a) Blood pressure will increase markedly because vasodilatation mediated by the parasympathetic system can no longer occur.
(b) Moderate exercise will become impossible because the blood supply to the skeletal muscle can no longer be increased by any means.
(c) The resting heart rate will rise because there will be a marked increase in sympathetic activity throughout the body.
(d) Sweating will no longer take place when the body temperature is raised.

57 Muscarine:
(a) causes excitation of only parasympathetic ganglia.
(b) occurs naturally in the bodies of most animals.
(c) when injected into the circulation causes vasodilatation.
(d) is inactivated by cholinesterases.

58 Which one of the following drugs is an example of a muscarinic agonist?
(a) Atropine.
(b) Hyoscine.
(c) Carbachol.
(d) Nicotine.

59 Which one of the following is NOT an antimuscarinic drug?
(a) Hexamethonium.
(b) Atropine.
(c) Hyoscine.
(d) Propantheline.

60 Eserine, an inhibitor of cholinesterase, reverses neuromuscular paralysis produced by curare by:
(a) competing for acetylcholine receptors in the postsynaptic membrane.
(b) depolarizing the postsynaptic membrane.
(c) prolonging the duration of acetylcholine in the synaptic cleft.
(d) causing the presynaptic terminal to release more acetylcholine per nerve impulse.

61 Eserine, an inhibitor of cholinesterase, can:
(a) also activate muscarinic receptors.
(b) also block nicotinic receptors.
(c) cause skeletal muscle paralysis as a result of acetylcholine accumulation.
(d) also slow the inactivation of noradrenaline.

62 Neuromuscular paralysis produced by decamethonium (C_{10}) cannot be reversed by eserine because:
(a) C_{10} cannot be displaced from nicotinic receptors by acetylcholine.
(b) the muscle endplate region is already depolarized.
(c) C_{10} produces neuromuscular paralysis by preventing the generation of nerve action potentials.
(d) eserine only facilitates the hydrolysis of curare.

63 Which one of the following does NOT enhance the effects of catecholamines?
(a) Thymoxamine.
(b) Pargyline.
(c) Cocaine.
(d) Desmethylimipramine.

64 The inhibitory effect of catecholamines on the Finkelman preparation is:
(a) only observed in the absence of calcium ions.
(b) typical of most smooth muscle preparations.
(c) caused by stimulation of α- and β-adrenergic receptors.
(d) caused by stimulation of muscarinic receptors.

65 Curare blocks conduction both at autonomic ganglia and at the neuromuscular junction because it:
(a) has both anti-muscarinic and anti-nicotinic properties.
(b) blocks cholinesterase.
(c) competes with acetylcholine for receptors on the postsynaptic membrane.
(d) depolarizes the postsynaptic membrane.

Autonomic nervous system

66 You would expect an increase in the extracellular potassium concentration to reverse the neuromuscular paralysis produced by curare by:
(a) competing for acetylcholine receptors in the postsynaptic membrane.
(b) depolarizing the postsynaptic membrane.
(c) prolonging the duration of acetylcholine in the synaptic cleft.
(d) decreasing the amount of acetylcholine released per nerve impulse.

67 If an animal was treated with an anticholinesterase drug, which one of the following symptoms does NOT appear?
(a) Dilatation of the pupil.
(b) Excessive salivation.
(c) Slowing of the heart.
(d) Increased gastrointestinal motility.

68 Which one of the following drugs increases the effect of cholinergic nerve stimulation?
(a) Neostigmine.
(b) Hexamethonium.
(c) Atropine.
(d) Curare.

69 Which statement is INCORRECT? Reserpine:
(a) decreases the binding of noradrenaline in the storage granules.
(b) antagonizes the action of tetramethylammonium.
(c) prevents granular uptake of dopamine.
(d) increases destruction of noradrenaline by mitochondrial monoamine oxidase.

70 Which one of the following substances would NOT stimulate the isolated heart from a reserpinized rabbit?
(a) Noradrenaline.
(b) Amphetamine.
(c) Isoprenaline.
(d) Calcium chloride.

71 Which statement is INCORRECT?
(a) Hemicholinium decreases the synthesis of acetylcholine.
(b) Triethylcholine decreases the storage of acetylcholine.
(c) Botulinum toxin prevents release of acetylcholine.
(d) Increasing the extracellular magnesium concentration decreases transmitter release.

72 Which statement is INCORRECT?
(a) Black Widow Spider venom depletes all nerve terminals of their stores of transmitter.
(b) Hemicholinium decreases synthesis of acetylcholine.
(c) Increased extracellular calcium concentration increases transmitter release.
(d) Neostigmine decreases the action of acetylcholine.

73 In an isolated preparation of rabbit ileum, which one of the following would inhibit the contractions?
(a) Eserine.
(b) Adrenaline.
(c) Acetylcholine.
(d) Carbachol.

74 The systemic blood pressure would be lowered following the administration of:
(a) noradrenaline.
(b) atropine.
(c) amphetamine.
(d) reserpine.

75 Giving hexamethonium to an intact animal would:
(a) lower its blood pressure.
(b) cause a depolarizing block of the skeletal neuromuscular junction.
(c) block the action of acetylcholine on the myocardium.
(d) block the α-adrenoreceptor.

76 Histamine:
(a) causes relaxation of intestinal smooth muscle.
(b) is a potent cardiac depressant.
(c) causes a marked increase in capillary permeability.
(d) causes contraction of skeletal muscle.

77 In an atropinized animal, the intravenous injection of which one of the following drugs would raise blood pressure markedly?
(a) Nicotine.
(b) Curare.
(c) Muscarine.
(d) Isoprenaline.

Autonomic nervous system

78 Stimulation of the peri-arterial nerves in a Finkelman preparation of rabbit ileum causes an inhibition of the smooth muscle. This inhibition can be blocked by:
(a) guanethidine.
(b) adrenaline.
(c) atropine.
(d) hexamethonium.

79 Which one of the following drugs would NOT inhibit the spontaneous contractions of isolated rabbit ileum?
(a) Noradrenaline.
(b) Adrenaline.
(c) Acetylcholine.
(d) Isoprenaline.

80 Which statement is INCORRECT?
(a) All sympathetic ganglia are stimulated by acetylcholine.
(b) The sympathetic nervous system releases only noradrenaline from its postganglionic terminals.
(c) Complete blockade of nicotinic receptors can cause death.
(d) Reserpine depletes stores of noradrenaline throughout the body.

81 Which one of the following treatments would block the sympathomimetic effects of amphetamine on the heart?
(a) Cutting the sympathetic supply to the heart one week previously.
(b) Cutting the vagus nerve one week previously.
(c) Hexamethonium.
(d) Atropine.

7 Gastrointestinal physiology

QUESTIONS

1 Which statement is INCORRECT? Salivary secretions:
(a) are enhanced by activation of the parasympathetic nervous system.
(b) are abolished by activation of the sympathetic nervous system.
(c) contain antibacterial agents.
(d) contain a higher concentration of K^+ than plasma.

2 The secretion of saliva:
(a) occurs in response to activation of the parasympathetic supply to salivary glands.
(b) is abolished by stimulation of sympathetic nerves.
(c) is primarily controlled by the presence of acid in the lower oesophagus.
(d) is essential for the initial stages of the digestion of lipids.

3 Which one of the following does NOT enhance the secretion of saliva?
(a) Sympathetic nerve stimulation.
(b) Parasympathetic nerve stimulation.
(c) Tactile stimulation within the mouth.
(d) Amylase.

4 The major enzyme of saliva is:
(a) trypsin.
(b) lipase.
(c) amylase.
(d) pepsin.

Gastrointestinal physiology

5 Which statement is INCORRECT? Salivary secretions:
(a) facilitate speech.
(b) reduce the occurrence of dental infections.
(c) produce chylomicrons in the mouth.
(d) contain an α-amylase.

6 Salivary secretions are abolished:
(a) during activation of the sympathetic nerve supply to the salivary glands.
(b) when weak acids are present in the mouth.
(c) at the onset of vomiting.
(d) by the administration of anticholinergic agents.

7 During swallowing:
(a) the smooth muscle of the upper oesophageal sphincter relaxes.
(b) non-adrenergic inhibitory nerves cause relaxation of the upper striated muscle.
(c) the lower oesophageal sphincter relaxes following activation of non-adrenergic inhibitory nerves.
(d) the striated muscle of the lower oesophageal sphincter relaxes following sympathetic stimulation.

8 During the peristaltic reflex in the small intestine:
(a) excitation of the circular smooth muscle layer precedes inhibition.
(b) only the longitudinal muscle layer is inhibited.
(c) excitation and inhibition of a given region of small intestine occur synchronously.
(d) none of these occur.

9 Which statement concerning the oesophagus is CORRECT?
(a) The upper portion of the human oesophagus contains a ring of smooth muscle.
(b) During swallowing the smooth muscle of the walls of the upper portion of the oesophagus relaxes during activation of the parasympathetic nerves.
(c) The smooth muscle of the lower oesophageal sphincter relaxes following the activation of non-adrenergic inhibitory nerves.
(d) The whole of the oesophagus is surrounded by an outer circular layer of smooth muscle.

10 Which statement concerning the musculature of the human intestinal tract is INCORRECT?
(a) The human oesophagus is in part composed of striated muscle.
(b) In the small intestine the smooth muscle adjacent to the serosa runs in the longitudinal direction.
(c) The external anal sphincter is under voluntary control.
(d) The colon contains only longitudinal muscle.

11 Which statement concerning the smooth muscle of the gastro-intestinal tract is CORRECT?
(a) The smooth muscle of the lower oesophageal sphincter contracts upon sympathetic stimulation.
(b) Gastrin relaxes gastric smooth muscle.
(c) Acetylcholine causes a marked relaxation of the small intestine.
(d) The external anal sphincter is composed entirely of circularly arranged smooth muscle fibres.

12 Skeletal muscle is to be found in the gastrointestinal tract of humans in all the following regions EXCEPT:
(a) lower oesophageal sphincter.
(b) upper oesophageal sphincter.
(c) external anal sphincter.
(d) upper third of the oesophagus.

13 Intestinal slow waves:
(a) result directly from the release of acetylcholine from the myenteric plexus.
(b) are propulsive contractions occurring along the small intestine.
(c) are initiated in the upper oesophagus by swallowing.
(d) are absent from the muscle of the upper oesophageal sphincter.

14 Intestinal slow waves:
(a) can only be recorded from ganglionic cells in the myenteric plexus.
(b) are rhythmic oscillations in the membrane potential of the smooth muscle cells.
(c) reach threshold for action potential generation only if the sympathetic nerves are stimulated.
(d) are generated by the pulsatile release of bile.

15 Non-adrenergic inhibitory nerves in the intestine:
(a) are responsible for receptive relaxation of the stomach.
(b) release acetylcholine on to the smooth muscle.
(c) release catecholamines on to the lower oesophageal sphincter.
(d) release Substance P on to the smooth muscle.

Gastrointestinal physiology

16 The basic electrical rhythm (slow waves) of the gastrointestinal tract:
(a) cannot be recorded from the muscle cells between meals.
(b) can only be recorded from neurones in the myenteric plexus.
(c) can control the occurrence of the contractions in the small intestine.
(d) are found mainly in the upper part of the oesophagus.

17 The basic electrical rhythm (slow waves) of the intestine:
(a) occur at a frequency of about 20 min^{-1} in the human stomach.
(b) occur only in the skeletal muscle of the upper oesophagus.
(c) are not present in the small intestine unless the tissue is contracting.
(d) occur synchronously with the segmenting contractions.

18 'Receptive relaxation' in the stomach is caused by:
(a) the release of acetylcholine on to the longitudinal muscle of the stomach.
(b) activation of the non-adrenergic inhibitory nerves.
(c) swallowing excessive quantities of air.
(d) an increase in slow wave frequency in the pyloric antrum.

19 Increased activity in the sympathetic nerves leading to the small intestine causes:
(a) more acetylcholine to be released from synapses in the myenteric plexus.
(b) less acetylcholine to be released from synapses in the myenteric plexus.
(c) excitation of the two smooth muscle layers.
(d) inhibition of the circular muscle layer alone.

20 Which one of the following does NOT initiate action potentials in the smooth muscle of the small intestine?
(a) The release of acetylcholine.
(b) Stretching a section of the intestine.
(c) Stimulation of the periarterial sympathetic nerve supply.
(d) The peristaltic reflex.

21 The spontaneous contractile activity of an isolated segment of rabbit ileum is due to:
(a) the rhythmic discharge of sympathetic ganglion cells in the serosa.
(b) oscillations of the resting membrane potential causing rhythmic bursts of action potentials in the smooth muscle.
(c) rhythmic activity from injured sections of the vagus nerve.
(d) the cyclic release of hydrochloric acid onto the mucosal cells.

22 Peristalsis in the small intestine:
(a) is caused by spontaneous activity of the vagus nerve.
(b) occurs due to the sequential activation of sympathetic nerves.
(c) is primarily controlled by the exocrine secretions of the pancreas.
(d) occurs following a local distending stimulus.

23 During the inhibitory phase of the peristaltic reflex, inhibition of the small intestine as a result of distension:
(a) is observed both above (oral) and below (aboral) the point of distension.
(b) is observed below the point of distension.
(c) is observed above the point of distension.
(d) results from increased activity of vagal fibres.

24 Peri-arterial stimulation (20 Hz, 1 ms, for 30 s) of the sympathetic nerves supplying the rabbit ileum (Finkelman preparation) causes inhibition of spontaneous contractions because they:
(a) stimulate non-adrenergic inhibitory nerves.
(b) release acetylcholine.
(c) release guanethidine.
(d) hyperpolarize the smooth muscle.

25 In the body of the stomach the mucosal cells secrete:
(a) gastrin, mucus and pepsinogen.
(b) hydrochloric acid, pepsinogen and mucus.
(c) hydrochloric acid and cholic acid,
(d) gastrin, intrinsic factor and vitamin B_{12}.

26 The parietal cells in the mucosa of the human stomach:
(a) inhibit gastric movements.
(b) produce nerve impulses.
(c) secrete acid.
(d) secrete gastrin.

27 During the gastric phase of the secretion of hydrochloric acid into the stomach:
(a) the concentration of H^+ in the stomach may be many million times greater than that in the plasma.
(b) the pH of the blood leaving the stomach falls.
(c) the secretion of intrinsic factor ceases.
(d) distension of the stomach inhibits the release of gastrin.

28 Which one of the following does NOT increase acid secretion in the human stomach?
(a) Vagal impulses.
(b) Gastrin.
(c) Atropine.
(d) Histamine.

29 During the cephalic phase of secretion of hydrochloric acid in the stomach, hydrochloric acid secretion:
(a) commences before food reaches the stomach.
(b) depends upon the intragastric concentration of gastrin.
(c) is increased by pancreatic lipase.
(d) depends upon the concentration of intrinsic factor.

30 Which one of the following does NOT reduce gastric hydrochloric acid secretion?
(a) Suppression of appetite.
(b) Acidification of the antrum.
(c) Vagal stimulation.
(d) Acidification of the duodenum.

31 Which one of the following stimuli does NOT lead to the release of gastric hydrochloric acid?
(a) Acetylcholine.
(b) Peptide fragments.
(c) Histamine.
(d) Fats.

32 Which one of the following events decreases the secretion of gastric hydrochloric acid?
(a) Release of gastrin from the antral mucosa.
(b) Smell of food.
(c) Activation of the vagus nerve.
(d) Distension of the small intestine.

33 Which one of the following is NOT associated with the intestinal inhibitory phase of gastric acid secretion?
(a) Release of secretin from the duodenal mucosa.
(b) Suppression of appetite.
(c) Presence of a high pH in the stomach
(d) Presence of acid in the duodenum.

34 Gastrin:
(a) is stored combined with the hydrochloric acid in parietal cells.
(b) is released into the bloodstream following distension of the pyloric antrum.
(c) is released into the lumen of the stomach by peptide fragments.
(d) causes marked inhibition of gastric motility.

35 Which one of the following is NOT contained in gastric juice?
(a) Intrinsic factor.
(b) Mucus.
(c) Pepsin.
(d) Acetylcholine.

36 The gastric emptying rate:
(a) is greater for fats than it is for carbohydrates.
(b) increases when the pH of the chyme leaving the stomach falls.
(c) decreases when the osmolality of the chyme leaving the stomach rises.
(d) is greater for proteins than it is for carbohydrates.

37 In the stomach, histamine:
(a) is located only in nerve cells.
(b) inhibits the actions of acetylcholine.
(c) is a biochemical precursor for the synthesis of gastrin.
(d) increases acid secretion.

38 If a compound diffuses passively through the stomach wall:
(a) that compound must be a weak acid.
(b) the total concentration of compound on either side of the stomach wall must be equal at equilibrium.
(c) the total concentration of compound on either side of the stomach wall must never be equal at equilibrium.
(d) the concentration of non-ionized substance will be equal on either side of the stomach wall at equilibrium.

39 A weak base is best absorbed from the small intestine because:
(a) the ionized form of the base can penetrate through the wall of small intestine.
(b) the pH of small intestine contents is lower than that of the stomach.
(c) the pH of the small intestine contents is higher than that of the stomach.
(d) active transport systems for the transport of all bases exist in the small intestine.

Gastrointestinal physiology

40 **In the colon:**
(a) the defecation reflex is activated by distension of the rectum.
(b) the secretion of pepsin promotes the absorption of amino acids.
(c) mass movements, occurring three times per day, return the contents of the colon to the terminal ileum.
(d) slow waves do not occur.

41 **Which statement concerning the colon is INCORRECT?**
(a) Distension of the rectal wall is the stimulus for defecation.
(b) Amino acids and glucose are actively absorbed from the colon.
(c) The active transport of sodium from the lumen results in the osmotic reabsorption of water.
(d) 'Mass movements' occur three or four times per day in the normal human colon.

42 **Ptyalin:**
(a) is secreted by the parotid gland.
(b) is most active within the pH range 1.3–4.0.
(c) is secreted by gastric parietal cells.
(d) cleaves peptide bonds in polypeptide chains.

43 **Pytalin is mainly involved in the digestion of dietary:**
(a) starch.
(b) cellulose.
(c) sucrose.
(d) glucose.

44 **Ptyalin:**
(a) is an α-amylase secreted by the parotid gland.
(b) has an optimum pH of 1.7.
(c) is secreted only in response to high circulating levels of gastrin.
(d) initiates the digestion of fatty acids in the mouth.

45 **During a meal the enzyme ptyalin:**
(a) is secreted primarily by the buccal glands of the oral mucosa.
(b) is active in the range pH 2–4.
(c) splits α-1,4-glucosidic linkages of starch.
(d) is secreted in a fluid with the same ionic composition as plasma.

46 **Which one of the following is NOT contained in chylomicrons?**
(a) Triglycerides.
(b) Secretin.
(c) Phospholipids.
(d) Free fatty acids.

47 Chylomicrons are likely to occur in large numbers in:
(a) lymph draining the intestine.
(b) the stomach.
(c) pancreatic acini.
(d) the intestinal lumen.

48 Which one of the following is NOT contained in micelles?
(a) Intrinsic factor.
(b) Phospholipid.
(c) Bile salts.
(d) Fatty acids.

49 Micelles are only 3–10 nm in diameter and consist of:
(a) bile salts, fatty acids, phospholipids and 2-monoglycerides.
(b) bile salts, fatty acids, and intrinsic factor.
(c) bilirubin, intrinsic factor and are 90% triacylglycerol.
(d) bilirubin, phospholipids and 50% triacylglycerol.

50 Glycocholic acid is:
(a) actively secreted into the duodenum by the pancreas.
(b) a bile acid released from the duodenal mucosa by a decrease in luminal pH.
(c) a bile acid found in micelles.
(d) a bile pigment formed from the breakdown of haemoglobin.

51 Secretin:
(a) is released into the duodenum by acid leaking from the stomach.
(b) causes parietal cell secretion to increase.
(c) stimulates the pancreas to release bicarbonate ions.
(d) is released into the terminal ileum by intrinsic factor.

52 Secretin:
(a) is the name given to the pancreatic juice.
(b) is a duodenal enzyme.
(c) stimulates production of alkaline pancreatic juice.
(d) is a pancreatic enzyme.

53 Cholecystokinin is:
(a) released by the cells of the antral mucosa of the stomach following acidification.
(b) a proteolytic enzyme released by the pancreas.
(c) a carrier for vitamin B_{12} in the intestinal tract.
(d) released by the duodenal mucosal cells in the presence of neutral fats.

54 Which one of the following does NOT increase parietal cell secretion?
(a) The sight and smell of food at the onset of a meal.
(b) An increase in the H⁺ concentration in the stomach.
(c) Gastric distension.
(d) The presence of peptide fragments in the stomach.

55 Which one of the following substances can be regarded as part of the exocrine secretions of the pancreas?
(a) Pancreatic lipase.
(b) Somatostatin.
(c) Glucagon.
(d) Insulin.

56 The exocrine secretions of the pancreas:
(a) include insulin and glucagon.
(b) are enhanced by sympathetic nerve stimulation.
(c) cause bicarbonate ions to enter the stomach and hence decrease gastric secretions.
(d) include an enzyme with similar properties to salivary amylase.

57 Which one of the following does NOT increase the exocrine secretions of the pancreas?
(a) Increased activity in sympathetic nerve supplying the pancreas.
(b) Cholecystokinin.
(c) Acetylcholine.
(d) Gastrin.

58 Which statement is INCORRECT? Bile:
(a) contains bile salts and bile pigments.
(b) emulsifies dietary lipids.
(c) is synthesized in the pancreas from cholesterol.
(d) is an excretory medium.

59 Bile is a mixture of secretory and excretory products. Which one of the following does it NOT contain?
(a) Cholesterol.
(b) Inorganic salts.
(c) Lecithin.
(d) Amylase.

88 Multiple Choice Questions in Physiology

60 Which one of the following acids would NOT be found in a conjugated form in bile?
(a) Cholic acid.
(b) Hydrochloric acid.
(c) Deoxycholic acid.
(d) Chenodeoxycholic acid.

61 Which statement concerning bile is INCORRECT?
(a) Bile salts are primarily formed from the breakdown of haemoglobin.
(b) Bile is concentrated in the gall bladder.
(c) Reabsorption of bile salts from the intestine leads to a further secretion of bile.
(d) Bile salts are required for the digestion of triglycerides.

62 Bile salts are:
(a) synthesized in the liver from cholesterol.
(b) secreted into the stomach from the common bile duct.
(c) conjugates of bile acids with hydrochloric acid.
(d) almost totally (95%) excreted from the body following a meal.

63 Bile salts are derived from:
(a) haemoglobin.
(b) glycerol.
(c) cholesterol.
(d) bile pigments.

64 Bile salts act:
(a) primarily to neutralize hydrochloric acid that leaks into the duodenum from the stomach.
(b) as carriers for the intestinal transport of amino acids.
(c) as carriers for the absorption of intrinsic factor in the colon.
(d) as emulsifying agents for large fat droplets in the upper intestinal tract.

65 Dietary carbohydrates are:
(a) predominantly digested within the acid medium of the stomach.
(b) digested in the mouth by α-amylase at a pH of 2.0.
(c) converted to disaccharides by α-amylase.
(d) all converted to fructose before absorption can occur.

Gastrointestinal physiology

66 Dietary carbohydrates are:
(a) primarily absorbed passively into the intestinal lymphatic system.
(b) often absorbed actively as monosaccharides from the small intestine.
(c) predominantly digested within the acid medium of the stomach.
(d) not digested by secretions in the mouth.

67 Dietary carbohydrates are:
(a) absorbed from the small intestine only if the pH is kept below 3.3.
(b) absorbed by a sodium-dependent process and transported to the liver via the lacteals.
(c) transported to the liver via the hepatic portal vein after breakdown to simpler monosaccharides.
(d) rapidly digested by enterokinase (enteropeptidase) in the duodenum.

68 Which statement about the absorption of proteins is INCORRECT?
(a) The gastric absorption of proteins is minimal.
(b) Most proteins are broken down to constituent amino acids before absorption.
(c) Many amino acids are actively transported by the intestinal mucosal cells.
(d) Pancreatic amylase converts proteins into polypeptides.

69 Which statement concerning the digestion/absorption of proteins is INCORRECT?
(a) Protein digestion cannot occur in the absence of acid secretion in the stomach.
(b) Carboxypeptidase splits off terminal amino acids from certain peptides.
(c) Many amino acids are actively absorbed by a mechanism that requires the presence of sodium ions.
(d) The gastric absorption of proteins is minimal.

70 Efficient absorption of fats in the alimentary tract:
(a) requires the presence of a pancreatic lipase.
(b) is facilitated by enterogastrone.
(c) is the principal function of the colon.
(d) occurs entirely in the form of free fatty acids.

71 The polysaccharide cellulose:
(a) is partially digested by bacteria in the colon.
(b) is dissolved by the hydrochloric acid within the stomach.
(c) is completely digested by the action of bile salts.
(d) acts to reduce the surface tension of droplets of fat in the small bowel.

8 Cardiovascular physiology

QUESTIONS

1. **Which statement concerning blood flow in the cardiovascular system is CORRECT?**
   - (a) The volume flow of blood in a large artery is the same as that in a capillary.
   - (b) The volume flow of blood in a large artery is less than that in a capillary.
   - (c) The velocity of blood flow in a large artery is the same as that in a capillary.
   - (d) The velocity of blood flow in a large artery is greater than that in a capillary.

2. **Blood flow is greatest through the:**
   - (a) inferior vena cava.
   - (b) coronary arteries.
   - (c) lymphatics.
   - (d) mitral valve.

3. **Blood flow (l min^{-1}) is greatest through the:**
   - (a) tricuspid valve.
   - (b) left common carotid artery.
   - (c) inferior vena cava.
   - (d) left and right renal veins (summed together).

4. **Blood flow is least through the:**
   - (a) brachial artery.
   - (b) pulmonary artery.
   - (c) mitral valve.
   - (d) tricuspid valve.

5 Blood flow in arteries is usually:
(a) laminar.
(b) frictionless.
(c) turbulent.
(d) steady.

6 The blood flow in a large artery is:
(a) proportional to its resistance.
(b) inversely proportional to its resistance.
(c) proportional to the fourth power of its resistance.
(d) inversely proportional to the fourth power of its resistance.

7 If the blood flow through an organ is being estimated by the rapid injection dye-dilution technique which one of the following is necessary? Measure the:
(a) concentration of the drug in the arterial blood.
(b) volume of blood contained within the organ.
(c) amount of drug extracted by the organ.
(d) concentration of the drug in the venous blood draining from the organ.

8 Blood flow velocity within the circulatory system is generally slowest in the:
(a) major veins, where pressure is relatively low.
(b) capillaries, where the very large number in parallel create a large cross-sectional area.
(c) pulmonary veins, because of the relatively low pressure within the pulmonary circuit.
(d) venules of the systemic circulation, because pressure is low and effective cross-sectional area is relatively large.

9 Which one of the following will lead to a decrease in blood flow?
(a) Increased driving pressure.
(b) Decreased resistance.
(c) Decreased haematocrit.
(d) Turbulent flow.

10 The resistance to blood flow of two vascular beds in parallel is:
(a) mainly determined by arterial pressure.
(b) more than if they were connected in series.
(c) the same as the resistance of the smaller of the two.
(d) less than the resistance of either bed alone.

11 The proportion of total flow energy as kinetic energy is greatest in the:
(a) aorta.
(b) arterioles.
(c) capillaries.
(d) vena cavae.

12 If the diameter of a glass tube conveying fluid is doubled, the resistance to flow will be multiplied by:
(a) 1/2.
(b) 1/16.
(c) 2.
(d) 16.

13 If one section of a blood vessel narrows down to half the diameter of sections on either side of it:
(a) the resistance per unit length of the narrow section will be eight times that on either side.
(b) the velocity of blood in the narrow section will increase in proportion to the reduction of cross-sectional area.
(c) the transmural pressure, i.e. pressure between the inside of the wall and the outside, will be greater in the region of constriction.
(d) because of the higher resistance of the narrow section, blood flow is less likely to become turbulent.

14 If the resistance of three 1 ohm resistors in series is compared with the resistance of three 1 ohm resistors in parallel, which statement is CORRECT?
(a) The resistance offered by each of the 3 ohm resistors is changed by connecting them in parallel.
(b) The resistance offered by each of the 3 ohm resistors is changed by connecting them in series.
(c) The overall resistance offered by the in-parallel resistors is less than that offered by the in-series resistors.
(d) The overall resistance offered by the in-parallel resistors is the same as that offered by the in-series resistors.

15 The equivalent resistance to three 3 ohm resistors in parallel equals:
(a) 1 ohm.
(b) 3 ohm.
(c) 9 ohm.
(d) 27 ohm.

16 Which one of the following does NOT determine resistance to blood flow?
(a) The degree of shortening of the smooth muscle in vessel walls.
(b) The geometry of the vascular bed.
(c) Blood viscosity.
(d) Arterial blood pressure.

17 The resistance offered to the circulation as a whole by the arterioles is greater than that of the veins because the:
(a) diameters of arterioles are greater than the diameters of veins.
(b) mean pressure in the arterioles is greater than the mean pressure in the veins.
(c) pressure drop from the beginning to the end of the arterioles is greater than the pressure drop from the beginning to the end of the veins.
(d) fluid which is carried away as lymph through the lymphatics has passed through the arterioles but will bypass the veins.

18 The resistance offered by 10 cm of brachial artery is:
(a) greater than the resistance of 10 cm of its smaller diameter branch, the radial artery.
(b) less in adults than in children.
(c) 16 times the resistance offered by a 5 cm length of the brachial artery.
(d) greater in anaemia (reduction in red blood cells) because of the increase in blood flow.

19 When the pressure in a sphygmomanometer cuff is slowly released the first sound to be heard results from:
(a) turbulent blood flow while the artery opens briefly at the peak of the pressure wave.
(b) closure of the aortic valves towards the end of systole.
(c) turbulent blood flow while the artery remains open, but narrowed throughout the arterial pressure wave.
(d) closure of the mitral valve early in systole.

20 If the pressure in a sphygmomanometer cuff is slowly released, the sound of the pulse will suddenly decline when:
(a) intermittent flow reduces turbulence.
(b) the atrioventricular valves open.
(c) blood pressure has fallen sufficiently.
(d) blood flow is continuous throughout the cardiac cycle.

21 Which statement concerning pressures in the cardiovascular system is CORRECT? The systolic pressure in the:
(a) pulmonary artery is less than the diastolic pressure in the aorta.
(b) pulmonary artery is less than the diastolic pressure in the pulmonary artery.
(c) aorta is less than the diastolic pressure in the pulmonary artery.
(d) aorta is less than the diastolic pressure in the aorta.

22 If the heart rate doubles while stroke volume is halved and there is no change in total peripheral resistance, mean arterial blood pressure will:
(a) fall.
(b) rise.
(c) show no change.
(d) rise or fall depending on the blood volume.

23 At rest, older subjects have a large pulse pressure due principally to:
(a) higher heart rate.
(b) higher stroke volume.
(c) lower arterial compliance.
(d) lower arterial resistance.

24 To use the Fick Principle to estimate cardiac output:
(a) it is sufficient to know the rate of oxygen consumption by the body and arterial and venous concentrations of oxygen.
(b) it is necessary to know arterial and venous concentrations of both oxygen and carbon dioxide.
(c) measurements of heart rate, cardiac oxygen consumption and coronary sinus blood oxygen concentration are needed.
(d) it is necessary to estimate the relative contributions by right and left ventricles.

25 In the normal circulation, the largest volume of blood at any moment is in the:
(a) heart.
(b) veins.
(c) capillaries.
(d) pulmonary vessels.

26 In a normal adult with a blood volume of 5 litres about:
(a) 3.5 litres are in the aorta, large arteries and arterioles.
(b) 1.5 litres are in the pulmonary circuit.
(c) 0.3 litres are in the capillaries.
(d) 0.15 litres are in the heart.

27 The blood volume can be estimated by measuring the:
(a) plasma volume and multiplying by the haematocrit.
(b) red cell volume and multiplying by the haematocrit.
(c) plasma volume and multiplying by 100/55.
(d) red cell volume and multiplying by 100/55.

28 Blood volume is monitored by:
(a) carotid sinus baroreceptors.
(b) carotid body chemoreceptors.
(c) bone marrow turnover receptors.
(d) low-pressure baroreceptors.

29 If a volume of blood approximately equal to one-third of the circulating volume is taken from an intact, conscious animal, an increase in heart rate will occur because:
(a) the heart has a smaller volume of blood to circulate.
(b) efferent vagal activity increases.
(c) the fall in blood pressure is detected by the carotid baroreceptors and this leads to vagal withdrawal, plus increased sympathetic activity.
(d) blood vessels in skeletal muscles will dilate due to increased activity in the sympathetic cholinergic dilator system.

30 The volume of blood in systemic veins tends to increase following:
(a) a decrease in venomotor tone.
(b) a decrease in blood volume.
(c) an increase in total peripheral resistance.
(d) an increase in heart rate.

31 Haematocrit is usually determined:
(a) gravimetrically.
(b) photometrically.
(c) by centrifuging a sample of blood.
(d) potentiometrically.

32 If the haematocrit is 30%:
(a) resistance to blood flow is decreased.
(b) capillary filtration pressure is decreased.
(c) whole blood viscosity is four times that of water.
(d) blood flow in the aorta is less likely to be turbulent.

33 Which statement is INCORRECT?
(a) Viscosity of the blood increases as the haematocrit falls.
(b) The resistance to blood flow in arterioles is proportional to blood viscosity.
(c) The rapid injection method of measuring blood flow uses a plot of log dye concentration against time.
(d) The continuous injection method is suited to measure blood flow through individual organs.

34 Evans blue injected into the bloodstream soon binds mainly to:
(a) plasma proteins.
(b) haemoglobin.
(c) water.
(d) red blood cells.

35 In determining the volume of extracellular fluid using Evans blue, samples are taken over a period of 40 minutes principally to:
(a) establish that mixing is complete.
(b) adjust for dissociation of the dye–protein complex.
(c) allow adjustment for loss of dye–protein complex from the bloodstream.
(d) allow statistical analysis of the results.

36 Which statement is INCORRECT?
(a) The total osmotic pressure of blood plasma is similar to that of 0.9% sodium chloride solution.
(b) The colloid osmotic pressure of plasma is about 25 mmHg.
(c) The total osmotic pressure of blood plasma is similar to that of 0.9% glucose.
(d) The colloid osmotic pressure of plasma opposes ultrafiltration of fluid from capillaries.

37 The left ventricle is thicker-walled than the right ventricle because it:
(a) has to eject a greater stroke volume.
(b) is the principal path of transmission of excitation from the sino-atrial node to the ventricles.
(c) must eject blood through a narrower orifice.
(d) has to do more work per stroke.

38 Papillary muscles:
(a) are vestigial structures.
(b) contain the natural cardiac 'pacemaker cells'.
(c) are part of the ventricular musculature.
(d) prevent the semilunar valves from everting during diastole.

98   Multiple Choice Questions in Physiology

39   When the heart is pumping at the normal rate, which statement is INCORRECT?
(a) The pressure in the arteries is greater than the pressure in the veins.
(b) The pressure in the right atrium is the same as the pressure in the left ventricle.
(c) The veins contain more blood than the arteries.
(d) A greater percentage of the blood is composed of plasma than of red blood cells.

40   The volume of blood within the heart is:
(a) greatest during systolic ejection.
(b) about 1 litre.
(c) increased during exercise.
(d) greatest just before ventricular systole.

41   The volume of blood flowing into the right atrium is on the average:
(a) less than that flowing into the pulmonary vein.
(b) greater than the flow into the aorta.
(c) the same as that flowing into the pulmonary artery.
(d) about 5 litres per beat.

42   Systemic blood flow continues during ventricular diastole because:
(a) atrial systole occurs during ventricular diastole.
(b) cardiac valves continually readjust blood flow throughout the cardiac cycle.
(c) the previous systole distends the arterial tree with blood.
(d) the sharp decline in venous pressure maintains the pressure gradient from arteries to veins.

43   The end-diastolic volume of the right ventricle is:
(a) increased during exercise.
(b) equal to the lowest pressure in the arteries during each beat.
(c) greater during inspiration than expiration.
(d) less than the end-systolic volume.

44   The end-diastolic pressure of the right ventricle is:
(a) about 80 mmHg.
(b) greater during inspiration than expiration.
(c) equal to the lowest pressure in the pulmonary arteries.
(d) less than the pressure in the small systemic veins.

45 The end-diastolic right ventricular pressure:
(a) is the maximum pressure normally found in the ventricles.
(b) occurs when the atrioventricular valves open.
(c) increases with increases in end-diastolic right ventricular volume.
(d) occurs just at the completion of passive filling of the right ventricle.

46. The atrioventricular valves:
(a) close as a result of contraction of the papillary muscles.
(b) close when the atrial pressure exceeds that in the ventricles.
(c) are made of smooth muscle which is spontaneously active.
(d) are closed during isovolumetric relaxation.

47 Opening of the atrioventricular valves:
(a) is heralded by the second heart sound.
(b) is due to the rise in pressure following atrial contraction.
(c) coincides with systolic ejection.
(d) is not due to contraction of the chordae tendineae.

48 In the cardiac cycle, closure of the atrioventricular valves occurs:
(a) soon after the first heart sound.
(b) at the beginning of the isovolumetric phase of ventricular contraction.
(c) just before the QRS complex of the electrocardiogram begins.
(d) when blood is ejected most rapidly from the atria.

49 During the phase of isovolumetric relaxation of the left ventricle the:
(a) left atrioventricular valve is open.
(b) pressure in the left ventricle is greater than the pressure in the aorta.
(c) venous return ceases.
(d) left ventricle volume was at a minimum at the commencement of this phase.

50 The period of maximum volume of the left ventricle corresponds approximately to:
(a) end of ejection phase of ventricular systole.
(b) end of phase of isovolumetric ventricular contraction.
(c) end of phase of isovolumetric ventricular relaxation.
(d) the middle of the P wave of the electrocardiogram.

51 Ventricular systole in a normal person:
(a) lasts about 30 ms.
(b) immediately precedes the phase of rapid filling.
(c) immediately precedes atrial systole.
(d) coincides with the P–R interval of the electrocardiogram.

52 During ventricular systole:
(a) 70–90 ml of blood is ejected from the left ventricle but only one-seventh to one-fifth of this volume is ejected from the right ventricle.
(b) 70–90 ml of blood is ejected from the right ventricle but only one-seventh to one-fifth of this volume is ejected from the left ventricle.
(c) the aortic and pulmonary valves open.
(d) the sinuses of Valsalva are refractory.

53 The aortic valves:
(a) open immediately ventricular contraction commences.
(b) only close following completion of ventricular contraction.
(c) remain open during diastole.
(d) open when ventricular pressure exceeds aortic pressure.

54 Purkinje tissue of the heart is primarily concerned with:
(a) rapid conduction of excitation.
(b) prolonged mechanical response of cardiac muscle.
(c) prevention of extra systoles.
(d) the timing of depolarization of the sino-atrial node.

55 The sino-atrial and atrioventricular nodes are:
(a) dense fibrous structures to which the four fibrous rings of the heart are attached.
(b) unusual in that, unlike other regions of the heart, they are not myelinated.
(c) excitable tissues.
(d) located in moderator bands.

56 Excitation of the ventricles of the heart:
(a) begins in the interventricular septum.
(b) is conducted to the ventricles from the atria via the chordae tendineae and papillary muscle fibres.
(c) does not occur when the Purkinje fibres are damaged.
(d) is limited to the special conducting tissues of the ventricles.

57 Rapid activation of all regions of the internal surface of the ventricles is achieved by the:
(a) sino-atrial node.
(b) atrioventricular node.
(c) Purkinje fibres.
(d) electrical continuity between adjacent cardiac muscle cells.

58 Which statement is INCORRECT?
(a) Increased sympathetic activity to the heart increases the rate of firing of pacemaker cells.
(b) Sympathetic stimulation can produce an increase in stroke volume by increasing the end-diastolic volume.
(c) Vagal stimulation has no effect on ventricular contractility.
(d) During inspiration blood flow into the right atrium increases.

59 Conduction of excitation from the atria to the ventricles in the mammalian heart:
(a) is via the sino-atrial node.
(b) is dependent on the presence of papillary muscles.
(c) can occur anywhere on the boundary between the atria and ventricles.
(d) is restricted to the atrioventricular node.

60 The cardiac action potential is conducted through the ventricular wall at about:
(a) $0.1\,m\,s^{-1}$.
(b) $1\,m\,s^{-1}$.
(c) $10\,m\,s^{-1}$.
(d) $100\,m\,s^{-1}$.

61 The cardiac action potential in mammals:
(a) is totally independent of the central nervous system.
(b) has a longer duration than a skeletal muscle action potential.
(c) is of the same configuration in atrial muscle and sino-atrial node.
(d) follows the Frank–Starling curve.

62 Cardiac contractility is said to be increased when:
(a) cardiac output increases without a change in heart rate or left ventricular end-diastolic pressure.
(b) cardiac output increases due to an increase in heart rate.
(c) cardiac output increases due to an increase in left ventricular end-diastolic pressure.
(d) the force–length curve for the ventricle is shifted to the right.

63 Which one of the following does NOT lead to an increase in cardiac contractility?
(a) Stroke volume.
(b) Firing of the vagus nerve.
(c) Firing of the sympathetic nerves.
(d) Firing of baroreceptors.

64 Denervation of the heart causes:
(a) failure of pacemaker activity in the sino-atrial node.
(b) failure of the grading of ventricular contraction in response to different degrees of filling.
(c) the resting heart rate to be faster because of the lack of vagal influences.
(d) cardiac slowing because of the lack of sympathetic influences.

65 Which one of the following does NOT contain a pacemaker?
(a) Duodenal muscle.
(b) Uterine muscle.
(c) Muscles that move the eye.
(d) Sino-atrial node.

66 The largest deflections in the electrocardiogram are most likely to occur when:
(a) ventricular depolarization is complete.
(b) a wave of depolarization is moving predominantly in a single direction in the myocardium.
(c) the bipolar leads are connected to the two arms and the wave of depolarization is moving caudally.
(d) there is a long delay between the QRS complex and the T wave.

67 The QRS complex of the electrocardiogram:
(a) occurs in different parts of the heart at different times.
(b) always occurs before excitation of the atrioventricular node.
(c) occurs while the aortic valves are closed.
(d) has the same duration as the ventricular action potential.

68 The QRS complex of the electrocardiogram:
(a) occurs in the atria before the ventricles.
(b) increases in amplitude with an increase in the end-diastolic volume.
(c) is widened with damage to the Purkinje cells.
(d) is recorded during ventricular contraction.

69 The QRS complex of the electrocardiogram coincides with:
(a) atrial systole.
(b) ventricular depolarization.
(c) ventricular repolarization.
(d) isovolumetric relaxation.

70 During the recording of the electrocardiogram, the P wave is:
(a) upward-going in lead II because the sino-atrial node is in the upper part of the right atrium.
(b) due to the depolarization of the sino-atrial node.
(c) smaller in complete heart block.
(d) only recorded in lead III when standing.

71 The P wave of the electrocardiogram:
(a) occurs during pulmonary valve closure.
(b) occurs during mitral valve closure.
(c) occurs during tricuspid valve closure.
(d) occurs during pulmonary valve opening.

72 In a normal adult person at rest, stroke volume is likely to be about:
(a) 7 ml.
(b) 20 ml.
(c) 70 ml.
(d) 400 ml.

73 The normal physiological cardiac output could be estimated by measuring:
(a) the output of the right ventricle and multiplying it by seven.
(b) into a volumetric vessel the initial flow from the freshly severed aorta.
(c) the output of the right ventricle.
(d) the arteriovenous difference in blood oxygen tension and dividing it by the oxygen consumption of the heart.

74 The mean cardiac output can be calculated directly from:
(a) mean heart size, blood pressure and heart rate.
(b) stroke volume and heart rate.
(c) peripheral resistance and blood viscosity.
(d) blood velocity and stroke volume.

75 **Starling's law is illustrated by:**
(a) a decrease in capillary hydrostatic pressure following vasoconstriction.
(b) an increase in cardiac contractility resulting from increasing firing of sympathetic nerves to the heart.
(c) an increased stroke volume resulting from an increase in end-diastolic pressure.
(d) the relation between end-diastolic pressure and end-diastolic volume.

76 **When the heart stops beating and the blood ceases circulating, which statement is INCORRECT?**
(a) The pressure in the arteries is greater than the pressure in the veins.
(b) The pressure in the right atrium is the same as the pressure in the left ventricle.
(c) The veins contain more blood than the arteries.
(d) A greater percentage of the blood is composed of plasma than of red blood cells.

77 **Blood travels to the head mainly via the:**
(a) jugular veins.
(b) azygos vein.
(c) carotid arteries.
(d) subclavian arteries.

78 **In performing Harvey's experiment to demonstrate the direction of flow in superficial veins of the forearm, a cuff is applied to the upper arm in order to:**
(a) raise the pressure in the veins of the forearm.
(b) lower the intravascular pressure in the arm distal to the cuff.
(c) prevent artefacts caused by arterial flow in the opposite direction.
(d) demonstrate that flow ceases when the veins are isolated from the heart.

79 **External compression of the carotid arteries between the heart and carotid sinuses leads to a fall in:**
(a) heart rate.
(b) systemic arterial pressure.
(c) respiratory rate.
(d) the frequency of vagal impulses to the heart.

80 External compression of the carotid artery between the heart and carotid sinus leads to an increase in the:
(a) stimulation of baroreceptors in the carotid sinus.
(b) sympathetic activity to the heart.
(c) parasympathetic activity to arterioles.
(d) end-systolic volume of the heart.

81 The timing of the diastolic pressure in the arteries corresponds approximately to:
(a) end of ejection phase of ventricular systole.
(b) end of phase of isovolumetric ventricular contraction.
(c) end of phase of isovolumetric ventricular relaxation.
(d) the middle of the P wave of the electrocardiogram.

82 In a normal adult the arterial:
(a) mean blood pressure is less than the arterial pulse pressure at rest.
(b) diastolic blood pressure is greater than the left ventricular diastolic pressure.
(c) pulse pressure is greater than the arterial systolic pressure during exercise.
(d) mean pressure is approximately equal to the arterial diastolic pressure plus one-third of the arterial systolic pressure at rest.

83 Among the consequences of increased arterial vasoconstriction to an organ is:
(a) a reduction in the amount of interstitial fluid in the organ.
(b) a reduction in that organ's contribution to the total peripheral resistance.
(c) a reduction in the difference in the oxygen content between the arterial and venous blood of that organ.
(d) an increase in the haematocrit of the venous blood of that organ.

84 The perfusion pressure along the brachial artery in the arm is:
(a) equal to the pulse pressure in the brachial artery.
(b) equal to the systolic pressure in the brachial artery.
(c) equal to the mean pressure in the brachial artery.
(d) proportional to the blood flow along the brachial artery.

85 Which statement concerning arterioles is INCORRECT?
(a) Blood velocity is greater than in capillaries.
(b) Mean pressure is less than in the aorta.
(c) The greatest change in pressure occurs here.
(d) Their walls are devoid of smooth muscle.

86   **Blood flow through arterioles:**
(a)   will be increased by an increase in activity in the sympathetic postganglionic nerves which innervate the smooth muscle of the arteriole.
(b)   is not subject to the control of the autonomic nervous system.
(c)   will be increased by a decrease in activity in the sympathetic postganglionic nerves which innervate the smooth muscle of the arteriole.
(d)   can only be altered by the precapillary sphincters where the capillaries branch from the arterioles.

87   **Which statement is CORRECT? The consequences of arteriolar vasoconstriction in an organ are likely to be a:**
(a)   decrease in capillary pressure in the vascular bed.
(b)   rise in blood flow through the organ.
(c)   fall in the level of products of metabolism in blood leaving the organ.
(d)   fall in total peripheral resistance.

88   **Arteriolar vasoconstriction in one particular organ is likely to lead to an increase in:**
(a)   capillary pressure of the organ's vascular bed.
(b)   the partial pressure of carbon dioxide in the blood leaving the organ.
(c)   the rate of lymph flow from the organ.
(d)   total peripheral resistance if the vasoconstriction is triggered by exercise.

89   **Precapillary sphincters are more likely to be open if:**
(a)   arterial baroreceptor firing decreases.
(b)   tissue oxygen consumption increases.
(c)   arteriolar vasoconstriction occurs.
(d)   tissue PCO_2 is low.

90   **The walls of vascular capillaries are thin and delicate but can withstand high intravascular pressures because:**
(a)   their wall tension is low as a result of their narrow diameter.
(b)   the interstitial hydrostatic pressure increases with the intravascular pressure, keeping transmural pressure constant.
(c)   there is a dense collagen network on the outside of the vessel.
(d)   blood velocity is very low in the capillaries.

91 Mean capillary pressure in the foot of a person standing motionless would be expected to be about:
(a) 15 mmHg.
(b) 25 mmHg.
(c) 35 mmHg.
(d) 105 mmHg.

92 Not much pulsation can be detected in capillaries because:
(a) capillaries are rigid tubes.
(b) capillaries are very compliant tubes.
(c) it is not possible to measure directly capillary pressure.
(d) most of the pulse energy is lost by damping in small arteries and arterioles.

93 Glucose is transferred across the capillary endothelium:
(a) by passive diffusion through intercellular pathways.
(b) by active reabsorption against a concentration difference.
(c) at a constant rate no matter what the concentration differences.
(d) to a greater extent the faster the rate of blood flow.

94 The normal central venous pressure:
(a) is about 25 mmHg.
(b) fluctuates with breathing.
(c) is normally below atmospheric pressure.
(d) is constant.

95 Haemorrhage of 10% of the blood:
(a) inevitably leads to death since adjustments by the cardiovascular system are unable to offset the loss.
(b) results in an increased haematocrit.
(c) leads to a rise in heart rate and fall in central venous pressure.
(d) is accompanied by a loss of fluid to the tissue.

96 Which one of the following is NOT increased following obstruction of a large vein (such as the inferior vena cava)?
(a) Vagal activity.
(b) Cardiac contractility.
(c) Arteriolar smooth muscle tone.
(d) Heart rate.

97 The venous pulse is:
(a) a damped arterial pulse.
(b) due to atrial fibrillation.
(c) due to smooth muscle contraction in the venous walls.
(d) partly due to respiration.

98 The flow of lymph is:
(a) about one plasma volume per day.
(b) equal to the cardiac output.
(c) equal to the capillary plasma flow.
(d) independent of plasma protein concentration.

99 The flow of lymph is:
(a) about one blood volume per day.
(b) increased when there is venous obstruction.
(c) increased when the arterioles are constricted.
(d) increased when the plasma protein concentration rises.

100 In which one of the following circumstances does oedema of the tissues NOT occur?
(a) Increase in arteriolar resistance.
(b) Increase in capillary hydrostatic pressure.
(c) Decrease in lymphatic flow due to obstruction.
(d) Decrease in plasma protein concentration of the blood.

101 Oedema may result if:
(a) arterial vasoconstriction occurs.
(b) plasma colloid osmotic pressure is raised.
(c) central venous pressure falls.
(d) lymph drainage is blocked.

102 Stimulation of baroreceptors in the carotid sinuses decreases the:
(a) vagal activity to the heart.
(b) sympathetic activity to the veins.
(c) volume of blood in the veins.
(d) interval between heart beats.

103 Stimulation of baroreceptors in the carotid sinuses:
(a) is decreased if the heart rate increases.
(b) is minimal at carotid sinus pressures greater than 200 mmHg.
(c) decreases the tonic sympathetic outflow to the heart.
(d) results in reactive hyperaemia.

104 Blood flows from the right to the left side of the heart through the lungs because the:
(a) systolic pressure in the pulmonary artery is less than the systolic pressure in the aorta.
(b) systolic pressure in the right ventricle is greater than the systolic pressure in the left ventricle.
(c) systolic pressure in the right ventricle is greater than the end-diastolic pressure in the left ventricle.
(d) blood is re-oxygenated in the lungs.

105 In comparison with the pulmonary veins, the pulmonary artery has:
(a) a lower transmural pressure.
(b) a lower content of carbon dioxide.
(c) a lower blood pressure.
(d) a lower content of oxygen.

106 During normal inspiration, the change in intrathoracic pressure results in:
(a) prolongation of systole.
(b) a decrease in peripheral resistance.
(c) no change in right atrial pressure.
(d) an increased venous return.

107 During prolonged exercise:
(a) the increase in cardiac output observed in largely brought about by the Starling mechanism.
(b) there is commonly a large rise in diastolic pressure.
(c) there is a fall in total peripheral resistance.
(d) mean arterial blood pressure remains at essentially the same value as at rest.

108 In exercise the flow of blood in active muscles:
(a) decreases because contraction of the muscles impedes the blood flow.
(b) decreases because the pulse pressure falls.
(c) increases because the pH in the muscles falls.
(d) increases because acetylcholine released from the somatic motor nerves relaxes the blood vessels.

109 In exercise the flow of blood in active muscles:
(a) is increased by the action of acetylcholine released at the skeletal neuromuscular junction.
(b) is increased because local vasodilatation occurs.
(c) falls because arterial pressure falls.
(d) is the same proportion of the cardiac output as it is at rest.

110 In which one of the following arterial parameters is there NO INCREASE during exercise?
(a) Systolic pressure.
(b) Diastolic pressure.
(c) Mean pressure.
(d) Pulse pressure.

111 Which one of the following does NOT increase during exercise?
(a) Mean blood pressure.
(b) Stroke volume.
(c) Venous oxygen concentration.
(d) Arteriovenous oxygen difference.

112 During mild exercise there is a decrease in:
(a) total peripheral resistance.
(b) arterial mean pressure.
(c) arterial pulse pressure.
(d) left ventricular end-diastolic volume.

113 Which statement best describes active hyperaemia? There is an increase in:
(a) blood flow to an organ due to its activity.
(b) blood flow to an organ after a period of insufficient blood flow.
(c) the red cell concentration in the blood in people who live and work at high altitudes.
(d) the red cell production in the bone marrow in people who live and work at high altitudes.

114 Active hyperaemia results from:
(a) a localized increase in blood pressure to promote an increase in blood flow to a particular organ or tissue.
(b) the increased haematocrit found in people who live permanently above 5000 m.
(c) an increase in blood flow to an organ or tissue after blood flow has been occluded for a period of time.
(d) an increase in blood flow to an organ, resulting from increased metabolic activity.

115 A person whose blood contains antigen B and antibody anti-A could safely receive a blood transfusion from a person whose blood group was:
(a) A or B.
(b) A or AB.
(c) O or B.
(d) O or A.

9 Respiratory physiology

QUESTIONS

1 **The direction of flow of water and blood across the gills of fish constitutes:**
(a) an open system for gas exchange.
(b) a cross-current system for gas exchange.
(c) a counter-current system for gas exchange.
(d) a pool system for gas exchange.

2 **Which one of the following functions CANNOT be performed by mammalian respiration systems?**
(a) Heat exchanger for thermoregulation.
(b) Filter system to protect systemic circulation.
(c) Continuous flow system for gas exchange.
(d) Metabolic organ for the activation and inactivation of hormones.

3 **Inspiration:**
(a) increases the venous return to the heart.
(b) is assisted by the surface tension forces in the alveoli.
(c) requires less muscular effort than expiration during quiet breathing.
(d) begins when intra-alveolar pressure increases above atmospheric pressure.

4 **The mean blood pressure in the pulmonary circulation is about one-sixth that of the systemic circulation because:**
(a) the volume of the pulmonary circulation is about one-sixth that of the systemic circulation.
(b) the resistance of the pulmonary circulation is about one-sixth that of the systemic circulation.
(c) the force of contraction of the right ventricle is one-sixth that of the left ventricle.
(d) the resistance of the left atrium is one-sixth that of the right ventricle.

5 Which statement is INCORRECT?
(a) Some of the smaller pulmonary vessels can be constricted during inspiration by expanding alveoli.
(b) The pressure in the pulmonary artery is always the same as that in the aorta.
(c) During sudden occlusion of the pulmonary artery, blood in pulmonary veins can provide the heart with a reservoir of oxygenated blood.
(d) The ventilation:perfusion ratio varies in different regions of the lung.

6 Which statement is INCORRECT?
(a) Airway diameter increases during inspiration.
(b) The flow of air is greater in the largest airways.
(c) The resistance to air flow is greatest at large lung volumes.
(d) The total diameter of the airway increases down the respiratory tree from the trachea.

7 Which statement is INCORRECT?
(a) During expiration, alveolar pressure is higher than intrapleural pressure.
(b) Airway resistance is decreased at high lung volumes.
(c) Air flow rate during passive expiration is directly proportional to pulmonary compliance.
(d) For a diver working at great depth, turbulent airway flow is more likely when breathing air–oxygen than a helium–oxygen mixture.

8 Which statement is INCORRECT? Respiratory dead space:
(a) saturates the air with water vapour before it reaches the alveoli.
(b) removes particulate matter from air before it reaches the alveoli.
(c) decreases during coughing.
(d) decreases during inspiration.

9 Which statement is INCORRECT? Physiological dead space:
(a) comprises both anatomical and alveolar dead space.
(b) is minimized by mechanisms which match air and blood flow to give a ventilation:perfusion ratio of 0.8.
(c) represents a variable fraction of tidal volume.
(d) is increased during expiration.

Respiratory physiology

10 The residual volume:
(a) represents the anatomical dead space and physiological dead space.
(b) is increased by breathing through a long tube.
(c) is maximal at the peak of inspiration.
(d) represents lung volume following a maximal expiration.

11 A complete expired breath of 1 litre contains 4% CO_2 and the last 10 ml expired contains 5% CO_2. From this it follows that the:
(a) residual volume is about 1500 ml.
(b) residual volume is about 800 ml.
(c) dead space is about 150 ml.
(d) dead space is about 200 ml.

12 A man breathes out fully, and then breathes from and into a bag containing 20 litres of O_2 only. After 12 breaths, analysis shows that the bag contains 1 litre of N_2 as well as some O_2. From this it follows that in this man the:
(a) dead space is about 150 ml.
(b) dead space is about 1 litre.
(c) residual volume is about 1 litre.
(d) residual volume is about 1250 ml.

13 The most important factor determining the tidal volume is the pressure difference between the:
(a) atmosphere and the intrapleural space.
(b) intrapleural space and the alveoli.
(c) atmosphere and the alveoli.
(d) oesophagus and the alveoli.

14 The following measurements are obtained on a patient:
Tidal volume = 500 ml;   Dead space = 120 ml;
Respiratory frequency = 15 min^{-1};   Cardiac output = 7 litres min^{-1}.
Which statement is CORRECT?
(a) The ventilation:perfusion (V:Q) ratio in this patient is normal.
(b) Alveolar ventilation is 6 litres min^{-1}.
(c) This patient is probably a child under 10 years of age.
(d) Ventilation:perfusion ratio is pulmonary ventilation divided by cardiac output.

15 Which statement is CORRECT? In a 70-kg normal male, the vital capacity divided by the tidal volume is approximately:
(a) 1/10.
(b) 1.
(c) 10.
(d) 100.

16   Which one of the following is CORRECT?
(a) Vital capacity = Inspiratory reserve volume **plus** Expiratory reserve volume.
(b) Dead space = Resting tidal volume **plus** Residual volume.
(c) Alveolar minute ventilation = Respiratory rate **times** (Tidal volume **minus** Dead space).
(d) Inspiratory reserve volume = Vital capacity **minus** Resting tidal volume.

17   In obstructive airway diseases such as asthma, the:
(a) vital capacity, but not the total lung capacity, is reduced.
(b) forced vital capacity, but not the forced expiratory volume in 1 s (FEV_1), is greatly reduced.
(c) forced expiratory volume in 1 s and the forced vital capacity are both greatly reduced.
(d) forced expiratory volume in 1 s is greatly reduced in comparison to the forced vital capacity.

18   The forced expiratory volume in 1 second (FEV_1) is increased by:
(a) constriction of the bronchi.
(b) adrenaline.
(c) histamine.
(d) acetylcholine.

19   Which one of the following lung volumes cannot be measured with a simple spirometer alone?
(a) Vital capacity.
(b) Functional residual capacity.
(c) Tidal volume.
(d) Inspiratory reserve volume.

20   A lung spirometer can NOT be used to measure directly the:
(a) respiratory frequency.
(b) oxygen consumption.
(c) total lung capacity.
(d) tidal volume.

21   Which statement is CORRECT? If part of the bronchial airway is obstructed, the:
(a) ventilation:perfusion ratio of the lung will be increased.
(b) ventilation:perfusion ratio of the lung will be decreased.
(c) total residual volume of the lung will be decreased.
(d) tidal volume will be increased.

22 **Which statement is INCORRECT? Gas flow through pulmonary bronchioles is:**
(a) reduced by increased carbon dioxide in pulmonary bronchioles.
(b) increased by lowering intrapleural pressure during inspiration.
(c) directly proportional to the pressure gradient between alveoli and atmosphere.
(d) inversely proportional to airway resistance.

23 **Which statement is INCORRECT? The conducting zone of the respiratory system:**
(a) contains goblet cells which secrete mucigen.
(b) contains alveolar ducts leading to alveoli.
(c) constitutes the anatomical dead space.
(d) does not take part in gas exchange.

24 **The conducting regions of the respiratory system:**
(a) contain alveoli at their branches.
(b) decrease in volume as the lung expands.
(c) contain cilia and mucigen for waste disposal.
(d) make up the physiological dead space.

25 **During quiet respiration, the alveoli at the base of the lung:**
(a) are better ventilated than those at the apex.
(b) remain fully expanded due to the effect of gravity.
(c) become engorged with tissue exudate.
(d) are less well ventilated than those at the apex.

26 **In a normal, healthy adult the alveoli remain free of fluid because of:**
(a) any remaining moisture being rapidly expelled by the cough reflex.
(b) the high arterial blood pressure in the pulmonary circulation.
(c) the colloid osmotic pressure exerted by plasma proteins.
(d) the action of surfactants to release the surface tension across alveoli.

27 **If a physiological dead space of 150 ml is increased by breathing through a tube of volume 500 ml, then with a tidal volume of 600 ml and a respiratory frequency of 16 min^{-1}, the alveolar ventilation rate is:**
(a) 5.6 litres min^{-1}.
(b) 2.4 litres min^{-1}.
(c) 8.0 litres min^{-1}.
(d) zero.

28
A man with an anatomical dead space of 150 ml swims using a snorkel with a volume of 90 ml. If he breathes 15 breaths min^{-1} and his tidal volume is 590 ml his alveolar ventilation will be:
(a) 5250 ml min^{-1}.
(b) 6600 ml min^{-1}.
(c) 7500 ml min^{-1}.
(d) 8850 ml min^{-1}.

29
Which one of the following does NOT occur when voluntary hyperventilation is sufficient to treble alveolar ventilation and is maintained for 2 minutes?
(a) The plasma proteins become more ionized.
(b) Total Ca^{2+} is unchanged but ionized $[Ca^{2+}]$ increases.
(c) A fall in plasma bicarbonate concentration in arterial blood.
(d) A brief period of apnoea immediately afterwards.

30
Which statement is INCORRECT?
(a) Alveolar surface tension facilitates alveolar–capillary gas exchange.
(b) Alveolar surface tension contributes to lung compliance.
(c) Breathing via a long tube increases respiratory dead space and tidal volume.
(d) Alveoli may collapse if surface tension is too great.

31
Which one of the following statements about the surface-active material (surfactant) lining the lung alveoli is CORRECT?
(a) The surfactant increases the surface tension of the film of liquid lining the alveoli.
(b) The surfactant decreases lung compliance.
(c) In the absence of normal surfactant there will be less tendency for alveoli to collapse.
(d) An indirect consequence of the absence of normal surfactant may be a fall in systemic arterial pH.

32
Intra-alveolar pressure:
(a) is always subatmospheric.
(b) is only subatmospheric during expiration.
(c) equals intrapleural pressure.
(d) equals atmospheric pressure at end-expiration.

Respiratory physiology

33 Which statement is INCORRECT?
(a) The alveolar–capillary membranes have a large surface area of 50–100 m^2.
(b) The small total thickness of the alveolar membrane aids diffusion of gases.
(c) A respiratory bronchiole may be distinguished from a terminal bronchiole by the alveoli budding from its wall.
(d) An erythrocyte spends 0.1–0.2 s in the pulmonary capillary bed during one transit in a resting subject.

34 Which statement is INCORRECT?
(a) Filling a lung with saline removes the air–tissue interface and hence the lung compliance is doubled.
(b) Laplace's law predicts that large alveoli should be expected to empty into small alveoli.
(c) The volume of blood in the pulmonary circulation is about one-sixth that in the systemic circulation.
(d) In mouth-to-mouth resuscitation, the alveolar pressure during inflation exceeds atmospheric pressure.

35 Which one of the following does NOT result from a deficiency of lung surfactant?
(a) Respiratory distress syndrome of the newborn.
(b) Difficulty in expanding the lungs.
(c) Air from small alveoli emptying into large alveoli.
(d) An increase in lung compliance.

36 The main factor which keeps the intrapleural space fluid-free is:
(a) positive atmospheric pressure acting on the chest wall.
(b) higher hydrostatic pressure in the pulmonary than in the systemic capillaries.
(c) surface tension between the parietal and visceral pleura.
(d) osmotic pressure of plasma proteins.

37 The pressure in the space between lung and chest wall becomes greater than atmospheric pressure:
(a) during a deep inspiration.
(b) during a cough.
(c) never in normal life because of the elastic tension in the lungs.
(d) when swallowing interrupts respiration.

38 Which statement is CORRECT? The intrapleural pressure becomes greater than atmospheric pressure during:
(a) deep inspiration.
(b) quiet expiration.
(c) attempted inspiration against a closed glottis.
(d) attempted expiration against a closed glottis.

39 During quiet respiration, which one of the following statements is INCORRECT?
(a) The resistance to gas flow is greatest during expiration.
(b) The maximum alveolar pressure occurs during inspiration.
(c) The airways are narrower during expiration than during inspiration.
(d) Inspiration has a shorter duration than expiration.

40 During quiet respiration at rest:
(a) expiration is active because the alveolar surfactant considerably alters the surface tension.
(b) expiration is passive because the elastic fibres of the lung are entirely responsible for deflation.
(c) expiration is due to the activity of internal intercostal muscles.
(d) intra-alveolar surface tension partly determines that expiration occurs passively.

41 During most of a forced expiration, flow rate is mainly limited by:
(a) contraction of the chest wall.
(b) inertia of the chest wall.
(c) hysteresis of the alveolar surfactant layer.
(d) compression of airways.

42 During the initial part of forced expiration:
(a) intrapulmonary pressure rises.
(b) intrathoracic pressure falls.
(c) intra-abdominal pressure falls.
(d) bronchial air flow rate falls.

43 Pulmonary compliance:
(a) is a measure of the rate of respiration.
(b) is reduced by pulmonary fibrosis.
(c) is measured in cm $H_2O\,ml^{-1}$.
(d) varies inversely with chest wall compliance.

44 Compliance of the lungs is:
(a) equal to the volume change in the lungs per unit change in transpulmonary pressure.
(b) equal to the change in intrapleural pressure per unit change in intra-alveolar pressure.
(c) less than the total compliance of the lungs and thorax.
(d) normally about 1 litre cm^{-1} of water.

45 The major muscle(s) active during forced expiration is (are):
(a) the diaphragm.
(b) the internal intercostal muscles.
(c) the abdominal muscles.
(d) the gluteus maximus.

46 Which statement about the function of the diaphragm is CORRECT?
(a) Its contraction causes a lowering of intrathoracic pressure.
(b) It is used during active inspiration and expiration.
(c) Its contraction causes expulsion of air from the lungs.
(d) Its contraction cases the intercostal muscles to relax.

47 In resting conditions the diaphragm is the major muscle of inspiration because it:
(a) shortens actively during inspiration.
(b) lengthens passively during expiration.
(c) contributes about two-thirds of the tidal volume.
(d) causes subatmospheric intra-alveolar pressure.

48 If a hole is made in the chest wall the thorax adopts a:
(a) deflated position because the intrapleural pressure is lower than normal.
(b) hyperinflated position because the pressure in the pleural space is lower than normal.
(c) hyperinflated position because the pressure in the pleural space is higher than normal.
(d) deflated position because the intrapleural pressure is higher than normal.

49 The goblet cells in the respiratory bronchi:
(a) secrete surfactant.
(b) secrete mucigen.
(c) engulf dust particles.
(d) produce cilia.

50 The most important reason why pulmonary diffusing capacity is usually measured with CO, rather than with O_2 or CO_2, is that:
(a) CO has a lower molecular weight.
(b) CO is much more soluble in aqueous media.
(c) people never have any CO in their blood when they come for the test.
(d) haemoglobin has a much higher affinity for CO.

51 Pulmonary diffusing capacity is:
(a) greater for oxygen than for carbon dioxide.
(b) defined as the volume of gas diffusing per mmHg per minute.
(c) increased by increased alveolar interstitial fluid.
(d) determined by the alveolar–capillary gradient of partial pressure.

52 Acclimatization to high altitude:
(a) is associated with the excretion of bicarbonate.
(b) requires that breathing rate increases to blow off more CO_2 in the lungs.
(c) requires a reduction in the number of red blood cells.
(d) is slowed by exercise.

53 In humans, during acclimatization to a high altitude (say 3000 m) over several weeks:
(a) physiological respiratory reserve decreases.
(b) blood haemoglobin concentration increases.
(c) arterial PO_2 increases.
(d) vital capacity decreases.

54 When a lowlander moves to high altitudes for several days, which one of the following does NOT occur?
(a) The pH of cerebrospinal fluid (CSF) first rises as the PCO_2 in CSF falls.
(b) Hypoxia stimulates peripheral chemoreceptors and hyperventilation occurs.
(c) The CSF bicarbonate rises and the pH returns to normal.
(d) Following an initial period of hyperventilation, eventual acclimatization is possible.

55 At high altitude, which statement is INCORRECT?
(a) Above 10 000 m the fractional concentration of O_2 in the alveolar gas is less than that of water vapour.
(b) Acclimatization to high altitude involves secretion of a hormone by the kidney.
(c) Medullary chemoreceptors become more sensitive to P_aCO_2.
(d) A subject could lose consciousness because hypoxia inhibits γ-aminobutyric acid (GABA) synthesis in the brain.

56 Analyses of gases in alveolar air and systemic arterial blood were made on a patient and were: alveolar air PO_2 = 102 mmHg; systemic arterial blood PO_2 = 60 mmHg. Based on these values which one of the following statements is CORRECT?
(a) These values are typical for a healthy person.
(b) They could be explained by a reduced diffusing capacity of the lung for oxygen.
(c) The values are typical for a healthy person who lives at high altitudes.
(d) The patient may have been hypoventilating.

57 A subject's functional residual capacity (FRC) was being measured by helium dilution. The initial and final concentration of helium in the spirometer were 10% and 6% and the spirometer volume was kept at 5 litres. The volume of the FRC was:
(a) 3.3 litres.
(b) 2.0 litres.
(c) 3.0 litres.
(d) 2.7 litres.

58 A shift of the oxygen dissociation curve of blood to the left:
(a) occurs in the pulmonary capillaries.
(b) is favoured by a rise in temperature of the blood.
(c) favours the passage of oxygen from blood to tissues.
(d) occurs in an anaemic person.

59 A shift of the oxygen dissociation curve of blood to the left:
(a) occurs in an anaemic person.
(b) occurs in a person exposed to carbon monoxide.
(c) is caused by an increase in the carbon dioxide content of blood.
(d) favours the passage of oxygen from blood to tissues.

60 Which one of the following does NOT shift the oxygen–haemoglobin dissociation curve to the left? A reduction in:
(a) temperature.
(b) pH.
(c) PCO_2.
(d) 2,3-diphosphoglycerate in the red blood cell.

61 Increasing hydrogen ion concentration causes the oxygen–haemoglobin dissociation curve to:
(a) become steeper throughout.
(b) become more distinctly hyperbolic.
(c) shift to the left.
(d) shift to the right.

62 Which statement is INCORRECT?
(a) The alveolar capillary membranes have a large surface area of 50–100 m^2.
(b) A red blood cell spends between 0.5 and 1.0 s in the pulmonary capillary bed during one transit in a resting subject.
(c) Oxygen diffuses approximately 20 times as easily as carbon dioxide through a liquid phase.
(d) The affinity of carbon monoxide for haemoglobin is approximately 200 times that of oxygen.

63 Myoglobin differs from haemoglobin in that:
(a) the myoglobin molecule lacks an iron–porphyrin complex.
(b) myoglobin has a greater affinity for oxygen.
(c) the oxygen dissociation curve for myoglobin lies to the right and below that for haemoglobin.
(d) myoglobin is not coloured.

64 The partial pressure of oxygen in normal arterial blood is approximately:
(a) 40 mmHg.
(b) 47 mmHg.
(c) 97 mmHg.
(d) 970 mmHg.

65 After breathing air at 10 000 m for 2–3 minutes, which one of the following would NOT show a decrease in the alveolar partial pressure?
(a) Carbon dioxide.
(b) Nitrogen.
(c) Water.
(d) Oxygen.

66 During a forced expiration air flow rate is NOT affected by the:
(a) size of the airways.
(b) elasticity of the lungs and chest wall.
(c) amount of turbulent flow in the airways.
(d) partial pressure of oxygen in alveolar air.

67 If a healthy subject hyperventilates with 100% oxygen for 2 minutes, then:
(a) apnoea will follow because there is no hypoxic stimulus to respiration.
(b) apnoea will follow because of an elevated arterial PO_2.
(c) apnoea will follow because arterial PCO_2 is reduced.
(d) the apnoea that follows will be of shorter duration than that following hyperventilation with air.

68 Alveolar carbon dioxide partial pressure would be increased by:
(a) decreased release of carbon dioxide from the blood.
(b) decreased ventilation of the lung.
(c) breathing pure oxygen.
(d) breathing 10% oxygen in nitrogen.

69 When carbon dioxide is taken up by blood perfusing active tissue it:
(a) mostly remains in solution due to its high solubility.
(b) combines with haemoglobin with a higher affinity than carbon monoxide.
(c) is mostly converted to bicarbonate ions in the red blood cells.
(d) causes chloride ions to leave the red blood cells as bicarbonate ions enter.

70 An increase in the carbon dioxide content of blood:
(a) reduces the partial pressure of oxygen.
(b) increases the capacity of haemoglobin to carry oxygen.
(c) moves the oxygen dissociation curve of haemoglobin to the left.
(d) favours the unloading of oxygen from haemoglobin.

71 Most carbon dioxide is carried in the blood in the form of:
(a) dissolved CO_2.
(b) HCO_3^-.
(c) H_2CO_3.
(d) carbamino compounds in the red blood cells.

72 When carbon dioxide is added to blood in the tissues:
(a) chloride shifts out of the red cell.
(b) oxygen is more firmly bound to haemoglobin.
(c) there is little change in pH partly because haemoglobin loses oxygen.
(d) the level of dissolved carbon dioxide in the plasma doubles.

73 If minute ventilation and CO_2 production remain constant, which one of the following will decrease the arterial PCO_2? Increase in:
(a) respiratory frequency.
(b) functional residual capacity.
(c) tidal volume.
(d) dead space.

124 Multiple Choice Questions in Physiology

74 In the sea, pressure below the surface increases by about 1 atmosphere for each 10 m increase in depth. A diver supplied with air at a pressure adjusted to that depth of 10 m is:
(a) breathing air in which the partial pressure of oxygen is 2.0 atmospheres.
(b) breathing air in which the partial pressure of oxygen is 0.4 atmospheres.
(c) breathing air with a higher nitrogen:oxygen ratio than at the surface and is therefore more prone to 'the bends'.
(d) getting a smaller amount of dissolved nitrogen when compared with levels at the surface.

75 Diving mammals are able to stay submerged for long periods because:
(a) during the dive they are able to drop their blood pressure sufficiently to minimize oxygen loss.
(b) during the dive they are able to reduce the blood supply to all but the vital organs.
(c) the measured myoglobin present in their muscles allows oxygen to be released to the tissues at higher partial pressures of oxygen.
(d) of a reflex acceleration of heart rate during the dive.

76 For deep-sea work at depths in excess of 100 m, helium is often substituted for nitrogen in the air supplied to the diver because it:
(a) stimulates metabolism.
(b) reduces airway resistance.
(c) distorts speech less, because of its lower density.
(d) diffuses more rapidly.

77 An engine mechanic is accidentally exposed to carbon monoxide which combines with half the haemoglobin in his blood. If he then breathes fresh air, which one of the following is INCORRECT?
(a) His alveolar gas PO_2 will be normal.
(b) His arterial blood PO_2 will be low.
(c) His arterial oxygen content will be low.
(d) His tissue fluid PO_2 will be low.

78 Mild carbon monoxide poisoning would lead to:
(a) increased arterial PO_2.
(b) decreased oxygen–haemoglobin affinity.
(c) increased alveolar PO_2.
(d) decreased arterial oxygen content.

79 **The peripheral chemoreceptors:**
(a) respond to an increase in arterial blood pressure.
(b) have a high blood flow per unit mass of tissue.
(c) are most sensitive to changes in PO_2 between 70 and 100 mmHg.
(d) are exquisitely sensitive to changes in PCO_2.

80 **The chemoreceptors that are particularly sensitive to pH are found in the:**
(a) major veins.
(b) medulla region of the brain.
(c) major arteries.
(d) pulmonary circulation.

81 **The carotid and aortic chemoreceptors:**
(a) monitor arterial oxygen partial pressure.
(b) monitor arterial carbon dioxide partial pressure.
(c) monitor arterial pH.
(d) have a blood flow, per unit mass, similar to that of the brain.

82 **The carotid and aortic chemoreceptors:**
(a) increase their rate of discharge when the PaO_2 falls below 80 mmHg.
(b) decrease their rate of discharge when the PaO_2 falls below 80 mmHg.
(c) decrease their rate of discharge when the PaO_2 rises above 40 mmHg.
(d) increase their rate of discharge when the PaO_2 drops to 30 mmHg.

83 **Carotid body chemoreceptors:**
(a) are rapidly adapting receptors.
(b) cease firing if the carotid arteries are occluded.
(c) increase their discharge as the PCO_2 of the arterial blood rises.
(d) are involved in the regulation of respiration.

84 **Chloride enters the red cell as oxygen is unloaded because:**
(a) it replaces the bicarbonate that leaves the red cell.
(b) reduced haemoglobin binds chloride more avidly than bicarbonate.
(c) haemoglobin catalyses the formation of $COCl_2$.
(d) active transport of chloride is facilitated by reduced pH and elevated PCO_2.

85 **In peripheral tissues, chloride ions:**
(a) diffuse into red blood cells as bicarbonate ions diffuse out.
(b) are actively pumped into red blood cells as bicarbonate ions are actively pumped out.
(c) diffuse out of red blood cells as bicarbonate ions diffuse in.
(d) diffuse into red blood cells as bicarbonate ions are actively pumped out.

86   **Which statement is CORRECT?**
(a)   Resuscitation is more often successful for drownings in fresh water than in sea water.
(b)   The central chemoreceptors are specifically sensitive to a change in $[H^+]$.
(c)   Oxygen is released by myoglobin at a higher partial pressure than haemoglobin.
(d)   During inspiration intrapleural pressure drops with a consequent rise in alveolar pressure.

87   **When a normal adult breathes a mixture of gases of composition 6% CO_2 : 94% O_2:**
(a)   respiration depth increases because of stimulation of medullary chemoreceptors.
(b)   respiration depth decreases due to increased vagal stimulation.
(c)   blood acidity drops because of an increase in respiration rate.
(d)   respiration rate increases because of the resultant hyperoxia.

88   **The neural control of breathing is exerted mainly by structures in the:**
(a)   pons and medulla.
(b)   hypothalamus.
(c)   spinal cord.
(d)   thalamus and cerebellum.

89   **Which statement about ventilatory reflexes is INCORRECT?**
(a)   Intercostal muscle spindles help to maintain ventilation when the lung compliance is suddenly altered.
(b)   Hering Breuer reflex is seen in adult humans only at high tidal volumes.
(c)   A hypoxaemic patient with some chronic CO_2 retention may develop a very high arterial PCO_2 when given 100% O_2 to breathe.
(d)   Increased body temperature, increased arterial PCO_2 and fall in arterial PO_2 all contribute to stimulating the increased ventilation on moderate exercise.

90   **When applying mouth-to-mouth respiration to a non-breathing patient, the chest may fail to rise. You should then:**
(a)   check that you are making an adequate seal and blow harder.
(b)   check that the airway is in the correct position and the seals adequate.
(c)   turn the patient into the coma position and extend the airway.
(d)   prop the patient up with blankets and seek help.

91 **A patient with pulmonary fibrosis would be expected to have:**
(a) a decreased lung compliance.
(b) an increased total lung capacity.
(c) a decreased FEV_1:FVC ratio.
(d) an decrease in FEV_1 and an increase in total lung compliance.

10 Renal physiology

QUESTIONS

1   Total body water:
(a) is a smaller proportion of body weight in men than in women.
(b) can be measured by the indicator dilution technique using tritiated water.
(c) comprises about one-third of body weight in young adults.
(d) comprises a smaller percentage of body weight in thin persons than in fat.

2   Intracellular water makes up:
(a) 15% of the total body water.
(b) 25% of the total body water.
(c) 55% of the total body water.
(d) 75% of the total body water.

3   The total osmotic concentration (osmolarity) of mammalian extracellular fluid is approximately:
(a) $3\,Osmols\,l^{-1}$.
(b) $30\,mOsmols\,l^{-1}$.
(c) $0.3\,Osmols\,l^{-1}$.
(d) $3000\,mOsmols\,l^{-1}$.

4   The concentration of K^+ ($mmol\,l^{-1}$) in mammalian extracellular fluid is approximately:
(a) 0.5.
(b) 1.0.
(c) 5.0.
(d) 10.0.

5   In the mammalian kidney which one of these fluids has the highest osmolarity?
(a) Glomerular filtrate.
(b) Plasma in the descending limb of the vasa recta.
(c) Interstitial fluid near the tips of the loop of Henle.
(d) Contents of the collecting duct, provided that antidiuretic hormone is absent.

6   The vasa recta of the kidney:
(a) pass into the medullary region, where they have a hairpin bend.
(b) carry blood in a nearly straight line from the afferent arteriole to the renal vein.
(c) lie almost entirely within Bowman's capsule.
(d) are highly convoluted blood vessels associated mainly with distal tubules.

7   Cortical nephrons (as distinct from juxtamedullary nephrons) in humans are found in:
(a) renal columns.
(b) medullary pyramids.
(c) major calyces.
(d) the renal sinus.

8   Renal clearance is measured as the rate of:
(a) urine formation divided by the renal plasma flow.
(b) excretion of a substance divided by the renal plasma flow.
(c) excretion of a substance divided by its systemic plasma concentration.
(d) excretion of a substance divided by its concentration in the urine.

9   The general Fick principle applied to renal handling of a plasma solute becomes identical with the equation for renal clearance if:
(a) the substance is completely filtered at the glomerulus.
(b) renal arterial concentration of the solute is zero.
(c) renal venous concentration of the solute is zero.
(d) adjustments are made for the presence of red blood cells.

10 The term 'renal threshold' is normally used to express a:
(a) urinary excretion rate.
(b) plasma concentration.
(c) urinary concentration.
(d) plasma clearance rate.

11 Renal filtrate differs from blood in that it lacks:
(a) ions and cells.
(b) ions and proteins.
(c) proteins and cells.
(d) ions and carbohydrates.

12 Which statement is CORRECT with respect to renal blood flow?
(a) Renal blood flow is greater per unit mass of tissue in the kidney medullary tissue than in the renal cortex.
(b) It is reduced during emotional stress.
(c) Its value is determined by the metabolic needs of the kidney.
(d) It is substantially increased during muscular exercise.

13 Blood flow through the kidneys in humans is about:
(a) 12.5 ml min^{-1}.
(b) 125 ml min^{-1}.
(c) 1.25 litres min^{-1}.
(d) 12.5 litres min^{-1}.

14 The afferent arterioles give rise to:
(a) glomerular capillaries.
(b) peritubular capillaries.
(c) vasa recta.
(d) efferent arterioles.

15 The pressure of blood within capillaries of the renal glomeruli:
(a) is lower than the pressure of blood in the efferent arterioles.
(b) increases when the afferent arterioles constrict.
(c) is greater than that in most other capillaries.
(d) decreases by 10% when arterial blood pressure falls by 10%.

16 Blood, having passed through the renal glomerular capillaries, passes directly into the:
(a) afferent arterioles.
(b) efferent arterioles.
(c) vasa recta.
(d) renal veins.

17 The glomerular filtration rate in a 70-kg adult male is normally about:
(a) 125 ml min^{-1}.
(b) 180 ml min^{-1}.
(c) 625 ml min^{-1}.
(d) 1400 ml min^{-1}.

18 A subject is given a drug which dilates the afferent arterioles. Glomerular filtration rate is consequently:
(a) unchanged because it depends entirely on the calibre of the efferent arterioles.
(b) decreased because the pressure at the end of the afferent arterioles is decreased.
(c) increased because of the lowered resistance to blood flow through the afferent arterioles.
(d) unchanged unless this drug causes a change in mean arterial blood pressure.

19 Glomerular filtration rate increases when:
(a) there is a decrease in the concentration of plasma proteins.
(b) the afferent arterioles are constricted.
(c) the ureter is blocked.
(d) the mean arterial blood pressure falls.

20 A positive component of the effective filtration pressure at the renal glomeruli arises from:
(a) glomerular capillary pressure.
(b) renal capsular pressure.
(c) osmotic pressure of plasma protein.
(d) pressure of urine in the bladder.

21 The normal glomerular filtration fraction in humans is approximately:
(a) 20% of cardiac output.
(b) 20% of urine production rate.
(c) 20% of renal blood flow.
(d) 20% of renal plasma flow.

22 Most of the water in the glomerular filtrate is reabsorbed in the:
(a) proximal tubule.
(b) loop of Henle.
(c) distal tubule.
(d) collecting duct.

23 The lumen of Bowman's capsule in the vicinity of the glomerular capillaries is lined with:
(a) macrophages.
(b) basement membrane.
(c) fenestrated epithelium.
(d) fenestrated endothelium.

24 The fluid obtained by micropuncture from the beginning of the proximal convoluted tubule contains:
(a) a concentration of sodium twice that found in plasma.
(b) a negligible amount of protein.
(c) abundant erythrocytes.
(d) a high concentration of renin.

25 The proximal convoluted tubules:
(a) reabsorb only a small proportion of the water and salts of the glomerular filtrate.
(b) contain juxtaglomerular cells which secrete renin.
(c) normally reabsorb all the glucose in the glomerular filtrate.
(d) are the main target cells for the antidiuretic hormone.

26 In the mammalian kidney, the loop of Henle plays an important role in the:
(a) control of antidiuretic hormone secretion.
(b) regulation of glomerular filtration rate.
(c) production of a concentrated urine.
(d) reabsorption of potassium.

27 The renal counter-current mechanism occurring in the loop of Henle is:
(a) one of the important instances where biological processes are not subject to the laws of thermodynamics.
(b) important for the maintenance of the interstitial fluid osmolarity in the renal medulla.
(c) responsible for Na^+/H^+ exchange in competition with Na^+/K^+ exchange.
(d) directly regulated by the circulating levels of antidiuretic hormone.

28 Appropriate units for transport maximum would be:
(a) $ml\,min^{-1}$.
(b) $mg\,min^{-1}$.
(c) $mg\,ml^{-1}$.
(d) $moles\,l^{-1}$.

29 Which one of the following renal processes is LEAST dependent on circulating hormones or neural reflexes?
(a) Na^+/K^+ exchange.
(b) Ca^{2+} reabsorption.
(c) Phosphate secretion.
(d) Diffusion of water across the ascending limb of the loop of Henle.

30 For which one of the following sets of hormones do all three hormones have major, direct effects on cells in the kidney?
(a) Antidiuretic hormone, aldosterone, adrenocorticotrophin.
(b) Antidiuretic hormone, renin, angiotensin.
(c) Adrenocorticotrophin, aldosterone, corticosterone.
(d) Antidiuretic hormone, aldosterone, parathyroid hormone.

31 Antidiuretic hormone is synthesized in:
(a) the hypothalamus.
(b) the granulated cells in the left atrium.
(c) the posterior pituitary.
(d) the macula densa and the afferent arteriole.

32 Antidiuretic hormone:
(a) is normally absent from the blood of conscious humans.
(b) if released into the blood, causes an immediate fall in blood pressure.
(c) increases the permeability of renal collecting ducts to water.
(d) is a most potent releaser of aldosterone.

33 Antidiuretic hormone is a:
(a) polypeptide hormone secreted by the posterior pituitary.
(b) proteolytic enzyme secreted by the juxtaglomerular apparatus.
(c) mineralocorticoid hormone secreted by the adrenal cortex.
(d) a prostanoid secreted by the efferent arteriole.

34 The signal which controls the secretion of antidiuretic hormone is:
(a) renin.
(b) the blood glucose concentration.
(c) the osmotic pressure of the blood.
(d) angiotensinogen.

35 Which one of the following would NOT be expected to increase antidiuretic hormone secretion by the posterior lobe of the pituitary gland?
(a) Injection of hypertonic saline in the carotid artery.
(b) Massive haemorrhage.
(c) Consumption of large volumes of water.
(d) Action potentials running along fibres from the supraoptic nucleus to the posterior lobe.

36 Which one of the following stimuli would lead to an increase in the secretion of antidiuretic hormone by the posterior pituitary gland?
(a) raised plasma osmolarity.
(b) lowered plasma osmolarity.
(c) ingestion of alcohol.
(d) positive sodium balance with negative potassium balance.

37 Angiotensin II:
(a) is a steroid hormone.
(b) is secreted by specialized cells in the kidney.
(c) has a direct action on the reabsorption of Na^+ by the distal convoluted tubule.
(d) is thought to have some vasoconstrictor activity.

38 The renal action of parathyroid hormone:
(a) directly regulates the filtered load of calcium ions.
(b) directly regulates the filtered load of phosphate ions.
(c) increases the excretion rate of calcium ions.
(d) increases the tubular reabsorption of calcium ions.

39 Renin is a substance secreted from cells in the:
(a) afferent arteriole.
(b) efferent arteriole.
(c) capillaries of the lung.
(d) liver.

40 Renin secretion would be promoted by:
(a) an increase in blood pressure.
(b) a decrease in blood pressure.
(c) an increase in the filtered load of sodium ions.
(d) an increase in the pH of blood plasma.

41 Which one of the following is the correct order of DECREASING renal clearance under normal conditions?
(a) Sodium, *p*-amino-hippurate, urea.
(b) Potassium, *p*-amino-hippurate, urea.
(c) *p*-Amino-hippurate, glucose, chloride.
(d) *p*-Amino-hippurate, urea, glucose.

42 At low arterial plasma concentration, the renal clearance of *p*-amino-hippurate is equal to:
(a) glomerular filtration rate.
(b) rate of excretion of *p*-amino-hippurate divided by its plasma concentration.
(c) body plasma volume divided by total renal plasma flow.
(d) renal clearance of inulin.

43 An osmotic diuresis can occur:
(a) only in the absence of antidiuretic hormone.
(b) despite the presence of antidiuretic hormone.
(c) only when glucose transport in the proximal tubules in unequal to the filtered load of glucose.
(d) whenever the counter-current mechanism is stimulated by aldosterone.

44 During an osmotic diuresis there is a marked decrease in:
(a) water reabsorption in the proximal tubule.
(b) urine volume.
(c) glomerular filtration rate.
(d) the renal clearance of *p*-amino-hippurate.

45 The diuresis associated with sugar diabetes is:
(a) an osmotic diuresis.
(b) a water diuresis.
(c) an antidiuresis.
(d) a pressure diuresis.

46 Which one of the following groups of words contains something of little importance to the renal handling of sodium ions?
(a) Adrenal cortex, lungs, liver.
(b) Aldosterone, renin, converting enzyme.
(c) Macula densa, active transport, afferent arteriole.
(d) Antidiuretic hormone, carrier-mediated transport, distal tubule.

47 The function of the proposed ionic counter-current multiplier system of the nephron is thought to be mainly:
(a) the exchange of cations for anions.
(b) the setting up of a gradient of osmotic concentration in the renal interstitium.
(c) increasing secretion of antidiuretic hormone.
(d) ensuring the secretion of a hypertonic urine.

48 The long-term regulation of hydrogen ion concentration in the body fluids is mainly dependent on:
(a) haemoglobin.
(b) plasma proteins.
(c) hormonal control.
(d) renal excretion.

49 In the kidney, carbonic anhydrase:
(a) occurs in the lumen of the proximal convoluted tubule.
(b) catalyses the reaction: $H_2CO_3 = H^+ + HCO_3^-$.
(c) plays an important role in the reabsorption of $NaHCO_3$.
(d) is essential for the reabsorption of glucose.

50 Of the following enzymes, the one most directly involved in reabsorption of $NaHCO_3$ in the proximal renal tubules is:
(a) carbonic anhydrase.
(b) converting enzyme.
(c) renin.
(d) the Na^+/K^+-ATPase.

51 The volume of extracellular fluid in humans can be determined using Evans blue dye:
(a) because Evans blue does not bind to proteins.
(b) by a single oral administration of the dye.
(c) if you assume the plasma volume to be a fixed proportion of the extracellular volume.
(d) because Evans blue is only found in the interstitial fluid compartment under equilibrium conditions.

52 Renal excretion of urea occurs mainly because of:
(a) active counter-current reabsorption of urea.
(b) acidification of urea with H^+ which causes it to be trapped within uriniferous tubules.
(c) passive diffusion of urea.
(d) secretion of urea in the middle third of the proximal tubule.

53 The renal clearance of inulin is an accurate measure of:
(a) renal blood flow.
(b) filtration fraction.
(c) urine flow rate.
(d) glomerular filtration rate.

54 **Inulin clearance in humans:**
(a) is determined by the capacity of the tubules to permit passive diffusion back into the plasma.
(b) is always greater than glomerular filtration rate.
(c) depends on plasma concentration of inulin, even if this is very low.
(d) is about 125 ml min^{-1}.

55 **If the clearance by the kidney of a substance X exceeds that of inulin:**
(a) X must be reabsorbed by the tubules.
(b) X is inert and is neither secreted nor absorbed.
(c) the concentration of X in the glomerular filtrate must be greater than the concentration of X in the plasma.
(d) X must be secreted by the tubules.

56 **Reabsorption of glucose from the renal filtrate occurs mainly in the:**
(a) collecting duct.
(b) loop of Henle.
(c) distal tubule.
(d) proximal tubule.

57 **In the normal human being, glucose appears in the urine when:**
(a) aldosterone secretion is elevated.
(b) the plasma glucose concentration is below the renal threshold for glucose.
(c) the glomerular filtration rate falls to zero.
(d) the rate at which glucose is filtered at the glomerulus exceeds the rate at which it is reabsorbed by the tubules.

58 **The normal plasma concentration of glucose is about 0.9 mg ml^{-1} and the renal clearance of glucose:**
(a) is normally about the same as that of inulin.
(b) exceeds that of inulin when inulin concentration is 0.9 mg ml^{-1}.
(c) approaches that of inulin when the glucose concentration is raised above 10 mg ml^{-1}.
(d) declines as glucose concentration approaches 2 mg ml^{-1}.

59 **If a certain substance X is found to be present in the urine, which statement is INCORRECT? X was:**
(a) filtered in the glomerulus.
(b) not filtered in the glomerulus but was actively transported into the urine.
(c) not filtered in the glomerulus but diffused passively into the urine as it passed down the collecting ducts.
(d) filtered in the glomerulus but was actively transported back into the blood at a rate which was slower than its filtration rate.

60 Most of the filtered load of water and solutes is reabsorbed in the:
(a) proximal tubule.
(b) loop of Henle.
(c) distal tubule when antidiuretic hormone is present.
(d) collecting duct when antidiuretic hormone is present.

61 The maximum possible osmolarity of urine in humans is:
(a) 60 mOsmolar.
(b) 280 mOsmolar.
(c) 1400 mOsmolar.
(d) 2800 mOsmolar.

62 The minimum concentration that can be achieved in human urine is about:
(a) 60 mOsmolar.
(b) 280 mOsmolar.
(c) 1400 mOsmolar.
(d) 2800 mOsmolar.

11 Endocrinology

QUESTIONS

1 Paracrine secretion:
(a) involves messenger substances bound to carrier proteins in the blood.
(b) involves the secretion of a substance to act locally without entering the circulation.
(c) involves secretion via ducts into the lumen of the gastrointestinal tract.
(d) never occurs in a normal healthy organism.

2 The pituitary gland:
(a) is essential for survival.
(b) controls the function of the parathyroid glands by a trophic hormone.
(c) is derived entirely from the roof of the embryonic pharynx.
(d) produces hormones all of which are peptides.

3 The vascular supply of the pituitary gland is of particular physiological interest because:
(a) it supplies only the neurohypophysis.
(b) substances carried in its blood control secretion of anterior pituitary hormones.
(c) its blood flows mainly from adenohypophysis to neurohypophysis.
(d) pituitary hormone secretion is controlled mainly by adjustment of its rate of blood flow.

4 The anterior pituitary:
(a) has a specialized portal blood supply.
(b) contains axons the cell bodies of which lie in the hypothalamus.
(c) produces prolactin in response to a releasing factor from the hypothalamus.
(d) function is unaffected by testosterone.

5 Secretory cells of the anterior pituitary gland are:
(a) known as acidophils and basophils.
(b) controlled directly by nerves from the hypothalamus.
(c) stimulated to secrete more adrenocorticotrophic hormone (ACTH) when corticoids are injected.
(d) of a single type which secretes at least six hormones.

6 Transplantation of the pituitary gland to a site remote from the hypothalamus would probably cause increased secretion of:
(a) oxytocin.
(b) prolactin.
(c) ACTH.
(d) melanocyte-stimulating hormone (MSH).

7 The hypothalamus:
(a) is synonymous with 'pituitary'.
(b) contains tissues that synthesize antidiuretic hormone (ADH) and oxytocin.
(c) lies ventral to the pituitary.
(d) has abundant neural connections with the anterior pituitary gland.

8 Which statement is CORRECT? The hypothalamic factors which regulate the release of the anterior pituitary hormones are all:
(a) primarily release-enhancing factors.
(b) small peptides of between 3 and 50 amino acids.
(c) secreted into the hypophyseal portal blood vessels.
(d) substances which are synthesized only in the hypothalamus.

9 Hypophyseal portal vessels:
(a) terminate at both ends in capillaries which lie in close association with secretory nerves.
(b) carry substances that affect the function of pituitary acidophils and basophils.
(c) are the sole source of blood to the posterior pituitary gland.
(d) most of the time carry blood up the infundibular stalk to the hypothalamus.

10 Hypophysectomy might be an appropriate treatment of:
(a) acromegaly.
(b) hyperparathyroidism.
(c) goitre associated with dietary iodine deficiency.
(d) male infertility.

Endocrinology

11 Which one of the following would be expected to increase food intake?
(a) stimulation of the lateral hypothalamus.
(b) anaesthesia of the lateral hypothalamus.
(c) stimulation of the ventromedial hypothalamus.
(d) hypophysectomy.

12 Antidiuretic hormone (ADH):
(a) is a large protein whose detailed structure is unknown.
(b) is rapidly released when neural impulses reach the posterior pituitary during water deprivation.
(c) by an indirect action, inhibits inflammatory reactions in tissues.
(d) acts principally through stimulating another endocrine gland.

13 Which one of the following would NOT be expected to increase ADH secretion by the posterior lobe of the pituitary gland?
(a) injection of hypertonic saline in the carotid artery.
(b) massive haemorrhage.
(c) consumption of a large volume of water.
(d) action potentials running along fibres from the supraoptic nucleus to the posterior lobe.

14 Which statement is INCORRECT? Vasopressin:
(a) is a potent vasoconstrictor.
(b) reduces the permeability of amphibian skin to water.
(c) enhances renal distal tubular water reabsorption in mammals.
(d) stimulates ACTH secretion.

15 The word 'oxytocin' is derived from words meaning:
(a) rapid birth.
(b) hormonal metabolite.
(c) acid secretion.
(d) respiratory poison.

16 Oxytocin and antidiuretic hormone both:
(a) are synthesized in hypothalamic cell bodies.
(b) are secreted by the adenohypophysis.
(c) are equally active in preventing a water diuresis.
(d) contain four sulphur atoms.

17 Which statement is INCORRECT?
(a) Oxytocin is synthesized in the suprachiasmatic nucleus of the hypothalamus and is transported into the posterior pituitary prior to secretion.
(b) Neurophysins are binding proteins for oxytocin and vasopressin which are co-synthesized and co-released with the two peptides.
(c) Vasopressin can both constrict blood vessels and promote renal water reabsorption.
(d) The hypophyseal portal blood system is unimportant in the secretion of oxytocin and vasopressin.

18 Oxytocin and prolactin both:
(a) have physiological actions on the mammary gland.
(b) are octapeptides.
(c) are steroids.
(d) are produced by the neurohypophysis.

19 In embryonic development, the adenohypophysis is derived from:
(a) the same precursor as the neurohypophysis.
(b) Rathke's pouch.
(c) an outgrowth of the infundibular stalk.
(d) the pars tuberalis.

20 Growth hormone:
(a) is secreted by pituitary basophils.
(b) increases the activity of the epiphysis in immature bones.
(c) is secreted independently of the hypothalamus.
(d) contains exactly 10 amino acids.

21 Which statement is CORRECT? Somatotrophin:
(a) stimulates the growth of cartilage via a mechanism involving the mediation of insulin-like growth factors.
(b) inhibits intracellular protein synthesis by both direct and indirect mechanisms.
(c) is a glycoprotein hormone consisting of two dissimilar subunits called α and β.
(d) when chronically hyposecreted by an individual leads to acromegaly.

22 Insulin-like growth factor is identical to:
(a) growth hormone.
(b) somatotrophin.
(c) somatomedin.
(d) somatostatin.

23 Prolactin secretion would be expected to increase following:
(a) transplantation of the pituitary gland.
(b) hypophysectomy.
(c) injection of hypothalamic extracts.
(d) injection of thyroid hormones.

24 ACTH:
(a) is a large protein whose structure is unknown.
(b) by an indirect action inhibits inflammatory reactions of tissues.
(c) is rapidly released when neural impulses reach the anterior pituitary during stress.
(d) has a structure which is identical with that of the melanocyte-stimulating hormone molecule.

25 ACTH has a chemical structure closely related to that of:
(a) melanocyte-stimulating hormone (MSH).
(b) prolactin.
(c) growth hormone.
(d) insulin.

26 Secretion of thyroid-stimulating hormone (TSH) would be expected to increase following:
(a) transplantation of the pituitary gland.
(b) hypophysectomy.
(c) injection of thyroid hormones.
(d) thyroidectomy.

27 Secretion of thyroid-stimulating hormone would be greatest when:
(a) the diet is deficient in iodine.
(b) secretion of ACTH is minimal.
(c) the adrenal glands are removed.
(d) thyroxine is injected.

28 Which statement about the function of the thyroid is CORRECT?
(a) Dopamine can cause release of a hormone which stimulates the growth of the thyroid.
(b) Thyroid hormone is mainly stored in secretory granules within the cytoplasm of the acinar cells.
(c) A chronic deficiency of dietary iodine leads to hypersecretion of thyroid hormone as a compensatory mechanism.
(d) The normal growth and function of the thyroid gland are dependent upon the presence of a functional pituitary and hypothalamus.

29 The thyroid gland is unusual among endocrine glands in that:
(a) its control is an indirect one, from the hypothalamus–pituitary.
(b) clinical conditions of both hypersecretion and hyposecretion exist.
(c) its products are temporarily stored outside the secretory cells themselves.
(d) its secretions are derived from amino acids.

30 Colloid of the thyroid gland:
(a) is found mainly in intracellular sites.
(b) exists largely as a store of extracellular thyroglobulin.
(c) is only readily detectable in hyperthyroid conditions.
(d) is a by-product of the breakdown of thyroid hormones.

31 Thyroid follicles:
(a) tend to be larger in diameter when stimulated by TSH.
(b) produce two chemically related hormones which have metabolic effects.
(c) have an epithelial lining three to four cells thick.
(d) store hormones loosely bound to a globulin by electrostatic forces.

32 Thyroid and ovarian follicles have in common that they:
(a) secrete steroid hormones.
(b) are small sac-like structures.
(c) are the sole hormone-secreting structures in the thyroid gland and ovary.
(d) are structures made up of a single layer of cells.

33 Calcitonin:
(a) is a molecule of exactly 10 amino acids.
(b) is secreted relatively independently of pituitary control.
(c) increases the activity of the epiphyses in immature bones.
(d) is secreted by pituitary basophils.

34 Thyroxine:
(a) is the only active hormone secreted by the thyroid gland.
(b) stimulates TSH secretion.
(c) is a breakdown product of TSH.
(d) contains exactly four iodine atoms per molecule.

35 Injection of thyroxine would be likely to cause
(a) increased output of thyrotrophin-releasing hormone.
(b) secretion by the crop gland of a pigeon.
(c) increased output of thyroid-stimulating hormone.
(d) increased metabolic rate.

Endocrinology

36 In relation to thyroxine (T_4), triiodothyronine (T_3):
(a) contains one less nitrogen atom.
(b) is a competitive antagonist.
(c) is more potent, weight for weight.
(d) is secreted in much larger amounts.

37 Triiodothyronine:
(a) has less biological activity, weight for weight, than thyroxine.
(b) contains exactly one nitrogen atom per molecule.
(c) is secreted as diiodothyronine which is then iodinated (to T_3) in the bloodstream.
(d) is more tightly bound than thyroxine to its carrier proteins in plasma.

38 The adrenal glands lie:
(a) cranial to the kidney.
(b) caudal to the kidney.
(c) lateral to the kidney.
(d) medial to the kidney.

39 Removal of the adrenal glands:
(a) would cause symptoms that could be entirely corrected by injection of small amounts of adrenaline and cortisone.
(b) involves removal of some tissue of neural origin.
(c) would prevent stress-induced changes in ACTH secretion.
(d) would be likely to lead to an increased Na^+ level in the blood.

40 Which statement about the adrenal gland is INCORRECT?
(a) Part of the adrenal is a modified form of sympathetic neuronal tissue which can secrete adrenaline and noradrenaline.
(b) Some hormones secreted from the adrenal gland can cause increases in heart rate and in the amplitude of heart beat.
(c) The chromaffin tissue in the adrenal gland is the main source of adrenaline in the circulation.
(d) None of the hormones that can be secreted by the adrenal gland is regulated by any pituitary hormones.

41 Which one of the following is NOT part of the adrenal gland?
(a) zona glomerulosa.
(b) zona reticularis.
(c) zona fasciculata.
(d) zona pellucida.

42 Adrenalectomy of a rat would be expected to:
(a) eliminate glucagon secretion.
(b) increase glucagon secretion.
(c) eliminate secretion of adrenocorticotrophic hormone.
(d) increase secretion of adrenocorticotrophic hormone.

43 Which statement about steroid hormones is CORRECT? They:
(a) always contain at least one nitrogen atom.
(b) are secreted by the adrenal medulla.
(c) have a three-ringed structure.
(d) have a chemical structure related to that of cholesterol.

44 All the major steroid hormones:
(a) have one or more double bonds in the A-ring of the molecule.
(b) contain 21 or more carbon atoms.
(c) are produced mainly by the adrenal glands.
(d) are more soluble in physiological saline than in lipid solvents like diethyl ether.

45 Steroid hormones act by circulating mainly as:
(a) free hormones and then binding to a receptor at the plasma membrane.
(b) carrier-bound hormones and then binding to an intracellular receptor.
(c) free hormones and then binding to an intracellular receptor.
(d) carrier-bound hormones and then binding to a receptor at the plasma membrane.

46 Which one of the following is NOT caused by secretion of inappropriate amounts of steroid hormones?
(a) Diabetes insipidus.
(b) Adrenogenital syndrome.
(c) Addison's disease.
(d) Cushing's syndrome.

47 Which one of the following is NOT a steroid?
(a) Corticosterone.
(b) Testosterone.
(c) Enterogastrone.
(d) Cortisone.

Endocrinology

48 Which statement is CORRECT? Cortisol:
(a) is inactive itself, but becomes active when oxidized to cortisone.
(b) is predominantly mineralocorticoid in action.
(c) increases the production of new glucose from amino acid precursors.
(d) has 17 carbon atoms.

49 Injection of cortisol would cause:
(a) a drop in blood glucose level.
(b) a drop in the number of circulating eosinophils and lymphocytes.
(c) an increase of ACTH secretion.
(d) a more rapid healing of wounds.

50 Aldosterone is mainly a:
(a) gonadal steroid.
(b) glucocorticoid.
(c) mineralocorticoid.
(d) gonadotrophin.

51 Which one of the following substances could be best described as a glucocorticoid?
(a) Androstenedione.
(b) Cortisol.
(c) Dehydrotestosterone.
(d) Corticotrophin.

52 Glucocorticoids such as cortisol or corticosterone:
(a) enhance glucose uptake by lymphatic tissue.
(b) antagonize the glycogen-depositing action of insulin in the liver.
(c) increase urinary nitrogen excretion.
(d) enhance the release of histamine by damaged cells.

53 The principal mineralocorticoid in humans is:
(a) corticosterone.
(b) 11-deoxy-corticosterone.
(c) cortisol.
(d) aldosterone.

54 Parathyroidectomy is likely to be fatal because of:
(a) an inability to regulate glucose.
(b) uncontrolled neuromuscular activity.
(c) renal failure.
(d) altered metabolic rate.

55 Which one of the following would cause a rapid rise in blood calcium levels?
(a) Removal of the kidneys.
(b) Removal of the parathyroid glands.
(c) Injection of parathyroid hormone.
(d) Injection of calcitonin.

56 Injection of parathormone causes:
(a) a fall in ionized calcium concentration in the plasma.
(b) decrease in renal tubular Ca^{2+} reabsorption.
(c) increase in renal HPO_4^{2-} excretion.
(d) antidiuresis.

57 Severe hypocalcaemia would probably cause:
(a) decreased secretion of calcitonin.
(b) increased secretion of calcitonin.
(c) decreased secretion of glucagon.
(d) increased secretion of glucagon.

58 Select the CORRECT statement. Islets of Langerhans:
(a) have long thin ducts to carry their secretions.
(b) secrete a fluid containing proteolytic enzymes.
(c) are found in the thyroid gland.
(d) contain α-cells and β-cells.

59 Select the CORRECT statement. Islets of Langerhans:
(a) consist of hormone-secreting cells embedded in tissues of the exocrine pancreas.
(b) are found mainly in the isthmus of the thyroid gland.
(c) contain the only pituitary cell-type with no known secretory function.
(d) are made up entirely of α-cells that secrete growth hormone.

60 Somatostatin is secreted by the D cell of the pancreatic islet into the interstitial fluid, from where it binds to a receptor on the β-cell and regulates insulin release. In this example, the somatostatin is acting as:
(a) an exocrine substance.
(b) an endocrine substance.
(c) a paracrine substance.
(d) an autocrine substance.

61 Proinsulin is converted to insulin by:
(a) chemical changes occurring in acinar cells.
(b) chemical changes occurring in blood.
(c) cleavage of a peptide chain from proinsulin.
(d) formation of new disulphide bonds.

62 Insulin:
(a) has an action on blood glucose levels opposite to that of glucagon.
(b) is given to patients suffering from diabetes insipidus.
(c) is secreted in larger amounts by the pancreas of a person suffering from diabetes mellitus.
(d) is a protein hormone whose amino acid sequence is unknown.

63 Secretion of insulin would be highest:
(a) during a fast.
(b) when pancreatic β-cells are congenitally absent.
(c) when glucose is injected intravenously.
(d) when there is a need to mobilize energy reserves into the blood.

64 Injection of insulin will cause:
(a) increase in plasma glucose concentration.
(b) increase in plasma glucocorticoid concentration.
(c) decrease in plasma free fatty acid concentration.
(d) decrease in plasma somatotrophin concentration.

65 An attempt is made to purify insulin from the pancreas using an initial extraction with an isotonic medium at neutral pH. It does not work because:
(a) the pancreas generally does not contain much insulin.
(b) the pH of pancreatic cells is low.
(c) the exocrine pancreas contains proteolytic enzymes.
(d) insulin requires the presence of other pancreatic substances for its hypoglycaemic action.

66 Which statement is CORRECT? Administration of an intravenous injection of human insulin to a normal rat will cause:
(a) an increased synthesis of glucose from glycogen.
(b) an increased synthesis of glycogen from glucose.
(c) a decreased synthesis of triglycerides.
(d) a decreased synthesis of protein.

67 Diabetes insipidus can be caused by a defect of the:
(a) anterior pituitary.
(b) hypothalamus.
(c) islets of Langerhans.
(d) acinar cells of the kidney.

68 Diabetes insipidus:
(a) could be induced by destruction of the appropriate hypothalamic nuclei.
(b) can usually be alleviated by the injection of insulin.
(c) is due to a defect of the anterior pituitary.
(d) causes high glucose concentration in the urine.

69 Ketone bodies are present in the urine during severe diabetes because:
(a) abnormal renal function allows ketosis to develop.
(b) lack of insulin allows the mobilization of excessive amounts of fat.
(c) diabetics have a distinct acidosis.
(d) ADH is required for normal metabolism of acetone.

70 Glucagon:
(a) acts by entering a target cell and binding to an intracellular cytoplasmic receptor.
(b) release is stimulated by acetylcholine.
(c) release is inhibited by adrenaline.
(d) acts by binding to a receptor on the surface of a target cell.

71 Negative feedback is NOT a major factor in the control of secretion of:
(a) ACTH.
(b) oxytocin.
(c) ADH.
(d) triiodothyronine.

72 Which hormone is synthesized in cell bodies of specialized neurones and released from their axon tips?
(a) Oxytocin.
(b) Growth hormone.
(c) Cortisone.
(d) Testosterone.

73 Which one of the following does NOT tend to raise levels of blood glucose in an otherwise normal animal?
(a) Injection of glucagon.
(b) Removal of the pancreas.
(c) Injection of an extract of adrenal medulla.
(d) Hypophysectomy.

74 Which one of the following would be most likely to cause the death of a rabbit as a result of hormone deficiency, if no corrective measures were taken?
(a) Adrenalectomy.
(b) Pancreatectomy.
(c) Thyroidectomy.
(d) Hypophysectomy.

75 Which one of the following words is the name of a single chemical compound, rather than a class of compounds?
(a) Mineralocorticoid.
(b) Thyronine.
(c) Oestrogen.
(d) Cortisol.

76 Which one of the following is the name of a single hormone rather than a class of hormones?
(a) Thyrotrophin-releasing hormone.
(b) Hypothalamic-releasing hormone.
(c) Mineralocorticoid.
(d) Glucocorticoid.

77 Which one of the following is a correct association of a gland, a hormone that gland produces, the chemical class of the hormone, and its action?
(a) Adrenal cortex – corticosterone – amino acid derivative – increases resistance to stress.
(b) Anterior pituitary – prolactin – protein – milk ejection.
(c) Neurohypophysis – vasopressin – cyclic peptide – dilation of arterioles.
(d) Parathyroid – parathyroid hormone – protein – increases removal of calcium from bone.

152 Multiple Choice Questions in Physiology

78 Which one of the following correctly associates an endocrine gland with the hormone it produces?
(a) Pancreatic islets – calcitonin.
(b) Hypothalamus – releasing hormone for luteinizing hormone.
(c) Anterior pituitary gland – corticosterone.
(d) Adrenal medulla – aldosterone.

79 Which one of the following correctly associates an endocrine gland with the hormone it produces?
(a) Pancreas – glucagon.
(b) Neurohypophysis – growth hormone.
(c) Anterior pituitary – corticotrophin releasing factor.
(d) Adrenal medulla – cortisol.

80 Which one of the following is the name of a single hormone rather than a class of hormones?
(a) Parathyroid hormone.
(b) Hypothalamic-releasing hormone.
(c) Glucocorticoid.
(d) Trophic hormone.

81 Which one of the following correctly associates a hormone with its major site of origin?
(a) Glucagon – acinar cells of the pancreas.
(b) Insulin – acinar cells of the pancreas.
(c) Aldosterone – zona glomerulosa of the adrenal cortex.
(d) Calcitonin – follicular epithelial cells of the thyroid gland.

82 Which one of the following correctly associates a hormone with its site of origin?
(a) Thyroid-stimulating hormone – follicular cells.
(b) Prolactin – anterior pituitary gland.
(c) Melanocyte-stimulating hormone – adrenal cortex.
(d) Growth hormone – thyroid gland.

83 Which one of the following is a correct association of a plasma constituent with a hormone that directly regulates it?
(a) Glucose – parathyroid hormone.
(b) TSH – thyrotrophin-releasing hormone.
(c) Na^+ – glucagon.
(d) Iodide – thyroxine.

84 Which one of the following correctly associates an endocrine gland with the name of an investigator well known for his study of that gland or its hormones?
(a) Neurohypophysis – Langerhans.
(b) Thyroid gland – Cushing.
(c) Ovary – Schally.
(d) Adrenal gland – Addison.

85 Which one of the following correctly associates a name with a scientific discovery?
(a) Banting – extraction of insulin from pancreas.
(b) Sanger – synthesis of growth hormone.
(c) Langerhans – effects of atrophy of the adrenal cortex.
(d) Du Vigneaud – development of the oral contraceptive pill.

86 Which one of the following is NOT a peptide or protein hormone?
(a) Triiodothyronine.
(b) Luteinizing hormone-releasing hormone.
(c) Calcitonin.
(d) Thyroid-stimulating hormone.

87 Which one of the following compounds is NOT an amino acid derivative?
(a) Noradrenaline.
(b) Melatonin.
(c) Triiodothyronine.
(d) Prostaglandin $F_{2\alpha}$.

88 Which one of the following correctly associates a hormone with its chemical structure?
(a) Oxytocin – peptide having a ring of 10 amino acids.
(b) ADH – large protein.
(c) Cortisol – 11-oxygenated steroid.
(d) Triiodothyronine – tripeptide.

89 Which one of the following correctly associates a chemical mediator with its site of origin?
(a) Renin – lung.
(b) Aldosterone – cells of the zona glomerulosa of the adrenal cortex.
(c) Growth hormone – acidophils of the pars intermedia.
(d) Thyroxine – parafollicular cells of the thyroid gland.

90 Which one of the following pairs contains the least-related chemical structures?
(a) Testosterone, oestradiol.
(b) Progesterone, cholesterol.
(c) Carbonic anhydrase, growth hormone.
(d) Glucagon, adrenaline.

91 Which one of the pairs includes two hormones least related to each other chemically?
(a) Growth hormone – prolactin.
(b) Aldosterone – oestrone.
(c) Oestradiol – testosterone.
(d) Parathyroid hormone – thyroxine.

92 Which one of the following has the greatest molecular weight?
(a) Adrenaline.
(b) Thyroxine.
(c) Thyroid-stimulating hormone.
(d) Corticosterone.

93 If we list sequences of hormones in descending order (i.e. highest to lowest) of molecular weight, which one of the following is INCORRECT?
(a) Oxytocin – insulin – ADH
(b) Renin – angiotensin – aldosterone
(c) Insulin – progesterone – oestradiol
(d) Growth hormone – insulin – thyrotrophin-releasing hormone

12 Reproductive physiology

QUESTIONS

1 **In meiosis the number of:**
(a) cells is doubled.
(b) cells is halved.
(c) chromosomes per cell is doubled.
(d) chromosomes per cell is halved.

2 **The anterior pituitary:**
(a) has a specialized portal blood supply.
(b) contains axons, the cell bodies of which lie in the hypothalamus.
(c) produces prolactin in response to a releasing factor from the hypothalamus.
(d) function is unaffected by testosterone.

3 **Feminine or masculine appearance is most directly dependent on:**
(a) the genotype.
(b) gonadotrophin output.
(c) hypothalamic factors.
(d) the level of circulating sex hormones.

4 **The normal delay in sexual development before puberty seems to be attributable to:**
(a) the high sensitivity of the hypothalamus to the feed-back effect of gonadal hormones.
(b) inability of the pituitary to produce gonadotrophin.
(c) failure of the gonads to respond to gonadotrophins.
(d) lack of effect of sex hormones on target tissues.

5   In which one of the following clinical states is the Y chromosome absent?
(a) Male mongoloid.
(b) Normal male.
(c) Klinefelter's syndrome.
(d) Turner's syndrome.

6   Luteotrophic action:
(a) is characteristic of substances called prostaglandins.
(b) refers to the fate of unruptured follicles.
(c) is shown by both prolactin and oestrogen in different species.
(d) prevents retention of spermatozoa in the epididymis.

7   The substance luteinizing hormone:
(a) is produced by the pars intermedia of the pituitary.
(b) is unimportant in reproduction in the female.
(c) could cause an increase in prostate gland weight if given by injection.
(d) causes adrenal cortical stimulation in males.

8   In a woman the amount of luteinizing hormone in plasma reaches a peak just:
(a) before ovulation.
(b) after ovulation.
(c) before menstruation.
(d) after menstruation.

9   Human chorionic gonadotrophin (HCG):
(a) acts to maintain the integrity of the endometrium during pregnancy.
(b) is produced in greatest quantity in the last 3 months of pregnancy.
(c) may be identified in the urine of pregnant women by an immunological technique.
(d) is a steroid hormone.

10 The administration of HCG to an ovariectomized rat results in:
(a) a reduction of uterine weight.
(b) an increase in uterine weight.
(c) proliferation of the endometrium.
(d) no effect.

Reproductive physiology

11 Injection of a purified preparation of follicle-stimulating hormone (FSH) into hypophysectomized rats would cause:
(a) follicular growth and copious oestradiol secretion in females.
(b) development of the seminiferous tubules in males and of the follicles in females.
(c) oestradiol secretion in females and testosterone secretion in males.
(d) gonadal atrophy in males due to a negative feed-back mechanism.

12 Hypophysectomy of a female rat would:
(a) cause atrophy of the uterus.
(b) block the effect of injected oestrogens on the uterus.
(c) cause an increase in FSH production.
(d) remove the source of luteinizing hormone-release hormone (LH-RH).

13 In a mouse, the greatest secretion of oestrogens occurs during:
(a) dioestrus and metoestrus.
(b) pro-oestrus and metoestrus.
(c) oestrus and metoestrus.
(d) pro-oestrus and oestrus.

14 The human ovaries:
(a) start to form ova at puberty.
(b) discharge 5–10 ova during each menstrual cycle.
(c) are essential for the cyclical activity of the uterus.
(d) release ova only if coitus has occurred.

15 Which one of the following treatments could NOT cause a reduction in the size of the right ovary of a rat?
(a) Hypophysectomy.
(b) Treatment with progesterone.
(c) Interruption of the hypophyseal portal supply.
(d) Removal of the left ovary.

16 Human ovarian follicles most commonly:
(a) are formed at puberty and survive several years.
(b) undergo atresia.
(c) ovulate and form corpora lutea.
(d) are lost at menopause.

17 Tertiary (Graafian) follicles can be distinguished from follicles at other stages in development by the presence of:
(a) granulosa cells.
(b) thecal cells.
(c) an antrum.
(d) an ovum.

18 Ovulation:
(a) in women is usually followed by a fall in body temperature.
(b) is best diagnosed by the rise in FSH that follows it.
(c) is triggered by impulses in the ovarian nerves.
(d) can be induced by injecting hormone obtained from pregnant women.

19 Following ovulation:
(a) there is a decrease in plasma progesterone levels.
(b) there is a decrease in basal body temperature.
(c) a secretory type of endometrium is formed.
(d) luteinizing hormone (LH) secretion begins.

20 Ovulation in the rabbit is distinct from ovulation in women because, in the rabbit:
(a) ovulation is induced by coitus.
(b) ovulation is always followed by pregnancy.
(c) luteinization depends on ovulation.
(d) ovulations do not alternate between left and right ovaries.

21 At ovulation the ovum enters the oviduct (Fallopian tube):
(a) by carriage in the bloodstream.
(b) by ejection directly from the follicle.
(c) because of the beating action of cilia.
(d) only if fertilization has occurred.

22 The ampullary region of the oviduct contains:
(a) a thin outer layer of circular smooth muscle and a highly convoluted epithelial lining.
(b) a thick outer layer of circular smooth muscle and a simple epithelial lining.
(c) a thick outer layer of longitudinal smooth muscle and a convoluted epithelial layer.
(d) no smooth muscle but a highly convoluted epithelial layer embedded in connective tissue.

23 The oviduct in a female mouse is:
(a) vestigial and has no physiological function.
(b) a short straight tube.
(c) absent.
(d) a tortuous thin tube.

24 Ovum transport through the oviduct:
(a) is of a similar time span in most animals.
(b) is brought about by the secretions of the luminal lining.
(c) requires that the ovum be fertilized.
(d) is independent of circulating steroid levels.

25 The presence of β-receptors on uterine smooth muscle cells:
(a) requires an intact sympathetic nervous system.
(b) may be modulated by the sex steroids.
(c) is assessed by the contractile response to noradrenaline alone.
(d) is detected by the contractile response to phenylephrine.

26 The myometrium:
(a) secretes prolactin.
(b) is not a target organ for progesterone.
(c) forms the maternal portion of the placenta.
(d) contains receptors for noradrenaline.

27 Contraction of the uterus:
(a) requires an intact nerve supply.
(b) is inhibited by the peptide oxytocin.
(c) may be modulated by the sex steroids.
(d) is caused by excitation of the smooth muscle membrane associated with the movement of Na^+.

28 The vaginal smear of a rat contains cells shed mainly by the:
(a) endometrium.
(b) ovaries.
(c) vaginal epithelium.
(d) myometrium.

29 In examining the vaginal smears of mice, the oestrous period would be identified by the:
(a) predominance of leucocytes.
(b) presence of round nucleated cells.
(c) predominance of cornified cells.
(d) absence of spermatozoa.

160 Multiple Choice Questions in Physiology

30 The vaginal smear obtained from a rat pro-oestrus is characterized by a predominance of:
(a) leucocytes.
(b) nucleated epithelial cells.
(c) keratinized epithelial cells.
(d) mucus.

31 The best explanation for the presence of leucocytes in the vaginal smear is that they:
(a) constitute part of the normal population of the vaginal wall.
(b) help dislodge the cornified layer.
(c) phagocytose debris.
(d) have no obvious purpose.

32 The best way to obtain a vaginal smear indicating oestrus in an ovariectomized mouse would be to inject:
(a) pregnant mare serum gonadotrophin .
(b) follicle-stimulating hormone.
(c) progesterone.
(d) oestradiol valerate.

33 In both the menstrual cycle of women and the oestrous cycle of other mammals:
(a) menstruation and ovulation occur at corresponding times of the ovarian cycle.
(b) the timing of sexual activity is determined by the same ovarian events.
(c) ovulation could be prevented by chronic treatment with progestagens and oestrogens.
(d) ovulation and menstruation occur when oestradiol levels are highest.

34 Which statement is CORRECT?
(a) Human chorionic gonadotrophin (HCG) is necessary for implantation.
(b) A fertilized ovum implants in the uterine wall within 24 hours of ovulation.
(c) Fertilization most often occurs in the oviduct.
(d) The placenta is formed solely by the mother.

35 Fertilization of the human ovum:
(a) normally occurs in the uterus.
(b) by one sperm normally prevents the other sperms from entering the ovum.
(c) occurs about 5 days after ovulation.
(d) occurs after implantation.

36 The corpus luteum:
(a) is maintained during pregnancy by prostaglandins.
(b) is formed only after ovulation has taken place.
(c) will form in the hypophysectomized animal if FSH is administered.
(d) is caused to degenerate by prolactin.

37 Corpora lutea are comprised mostly of:
(a) granulosa cells.
(b) interstitial cells.
(c) thecal cells.
(d) Leydig cells.

38 The maintenance of the human corpus luteum during early pregnancy is due to a hormone produced by the:
(a) chorion.
(b) endometrium.
(c) adenohypophysis.
(d) ovary.

39 Active destruction of the corpus luteum is:
(a) important in the regulation of the human menstrual cycle.
(b) accentuated by removal of the uterus.
(c) mediated by prostaglandins in some species.
(d) an important part of the actions of FSH.

40 The placenta:
(a) in the human produces hormones that affect the mammary glands.
(b) is unable to produce the same steroids as the ovaries.
(c) of the human differs from most other species in the many layers of tissue separating the maternal and fetal circulations.
(d) relies on maternal pituitary support throughout gestation.

41 In the placenta:
(a) there is mixing of maternal and fetal blood in the sinusoids.
(b) the PO_2 in the sinusoids is similar to that in the maternal alveolar air.
(c) the blood leaving the umbilical vein has a PO_2 similar to that in the sinusoids.
(d) the blood leaving the umbilical vein is about 70% saturated.

42 An assay for prolactin might make use of the fact that prolactin:
(a) causes myoepithelial cells of the mammary gland to contract.
(b) prolongs the functional life of corpora lutea in guinea-pigs.
(c) lengthens the interval between successive oestrous periods in rats.
(d) is secreted by the hypothalamus.

43 Progesterone is thought to reduce uterine contractions during pregnancy by:
(a) depolarizing the smooth muscle cell membrane.
(b) decreasing cell-to-cell coupling.
(c) blocking calcium entry into the smooth muscle cells.
(d) all of the above.

44 Normal parturition depends on:
(a) an intact autonomic innervation of the uterus.
(b) normally functioning ovaries.
(c) an intact posterior pituitary.
(d) dilation of the cervix.

45 Parturition:
(a) begins when the progesterone level reaches a critical maximum.
(b) cannot occur unless the neurohypophyseal system is intact.
(c) may be prolonged if the fetal anterior pituitary is impaired.
(d) may be prolonged by administration of catecholamines.

46 The formation of milk by the mammary gland:
(a) is stimulated by oestrogen and progesterone.
(b) ceases if the anterior pituitary is destroyed.
(c) ceases if the posterior pituitary is destroyed.
(d) is independent of afferent impulses from sensory receptors in the nipple area to the brain.

47 Cessation of reproduction in women is:
(a) called menarche.
(b) due to failure of the ovaries to respond to gonadotrophic hormones.
(c) due to senile changes in the hypothalamus.
(d) due to pituitary failure.

48 Castration in the male rat would result in:
(a) luteinizing hormone levels falling in the plasma.
(b) testosterone levels increasing in the plasma.
(c) seminal vesicle weight decreasing.
(d) prostate gland weight increasing.

Reproductive physiology 163

49 The formation of a testis from the undifferentiated gonad:
(a) is dependent entirely on the presence of a Y chromosome.
(b) is preceded by secondary sex cord formation.
(c) depends on Leydig cell activation.
(d) requires the presence of a functional Mullerian duct.

50 The testis fixed in the abdominal cavity in unilateral cryptorchidism:
(a) enlarges because of the increase in metabolism resulting from the higher temperature.
(b) is unaffected by the change in temperature because the appropriate testicular temperature is maintained by the pampiniform plexus.
(c) decreased in size because the increase in temperature interferes with spermatogenesis.
(d) decreases in size because the surgical procedure interferes with the blood supply.

51 The testicular cells responsible for secreting testosterone are:
(a) epididymal cells.
(b) Leydig (interstitial) cells.
(c) Sertoli cells.
(d) located within the seminiferous tubules.

52 Which is the CORRECT statement? Testosterone:
(a) levels in the circulation are maintained constant by feed-back stimulation of LH.
(b) is formed mainly in the lumen of the seminiferous tubules.
(c) is concentrated in the testis by the pampiniform plexus.
(d) enhances, but is not necessary for spermatogenesis.

53 Which is the CORRECT statement? Testosterone is:
(a) secreted packaged in seminal vesicles.
(b) responsible for the characteristic hair pattern of men.
(c) readily converted to aldosterone by the Leydig cells.
(d) not involved in spermatogenesis.

54 Which is CORRECT? Testosterone:
(a) is responsible for the reduced weight of the seminal vesicles after puberty.
(b) is excreted as an oxysteroid.
(c) is chiefly formed in the lumen of the seminiferous tubules.
(d) stimulates the production of pituitary gonadotrophin.

55 Spermatogenesis is NOT controlled by:
(a) secretion of testosterone.
(b) functional Leydig (interstitial) cells.
(c) secretion of FSH.
(d) a normally functioning vas deferens.

56 Choose the CORRECT statement. Spermatozoa:
(a) are produced at a faster rate when testicular temperature is raised to 37°C.
(b) are motile in the seminiferous tubules.
(c) normally contain 23 chromosomes.
(d) are stored in the prostate.

57 Adjustment of the temperature in the testis involves a counter-current heat exchange system in the:
(a) epididymis.
(b) vas deferens.
(c) pampiniform plexus.
(d) seminiferous tubules.

58 Erection of the penis:
(a) is associated with stimulation of vasoconstrictor sympathetic nerves to the penile arterioles.
(b) is associated with stimulation of vasodilator parasympathetic nerves to the penile arterioles.
(c) becomes impaired following vasectomy and this is apparently the result of a decrease in circulating testosterone.
(d) can occur following spinal transection at T12.

59 Which statement is CORRECT?
(a) Ejaculation of sperm does not require involvement of the sympathetic nervous system.
(b) During ejaculation seminal fluid is propelled out by rhythmical contractions of the skeletal muscles at the base of the penis.
(c) Erection is essential for ejaculation.
(d) Erection is associated with stimulation of vasoconstrictor sympathetic nerves to the penile arterioles.

60 Semen does not contain:
(a) buffers which help to neutralize the acid medium of the vagina.
(b) fructose.
(c) prostaglandins.
(d) sperm cells which have been stored in the seminal vesicles.

61 The greatest volume of seminal constituents comes from:
(a) bulbourethral glands and vas deferens.
(b) testis and epididymis.
(c) seminal vesicles and prostate gland.
(d) seminiferous tubules.

62 Vasectomy:
(a) involves removal of the prostate gland.
(b) prevents secretion of testosterone.
(c) prevents ejaculation.
(d) prevents neither secretion of testosterone nor ejaculation.

13 Answers

1 Cell physiology

1. a	2. b	3. d	4. d	5. b	6. d
7. b	8. d	9. c	10. a	11. b	12. a
13. d	14. b	15. b	16. d	17. b	18. a
19. b	20. d	21. c	22. c	23. b	24. c
25. c	26. d	27. d	28. c	29. b	30. c
31. c	32. b	33. d	34. c	35. b	36. d
37. b	38. a	39. a	40. d	41. d	42. b
43. d	44. d	45. a	46. b	47. d	48. a
49. c	50. b	51. b	52. a	53. d	54. c
55. a	56. d	57. a	58. d	59. d	60. c

2 Muscle physiology

1. d	2. d	3. b	4. a	5. c	6. d
7. a	8. c	9. c	10. d	11. a	12. a
13. b	14. c	15. c	16. d	17. a	18. a
19. c	20. c	21. c	22. b	23. c	24. c
25. d	26. c	27. a	28. c	29. a	30. b
31. b	32. c	33. d	34. c	35. d	36. d
37. c	38. b	39. c	40. d	41. b	42. c
43. c	44. c	45. b	46. b	47. b	48. d
49. d	50. a	51. b	52. d	53. d	54. b
55. b	56. c	57. d	58. b	59. b	60. a
61. c	62. b	63. a	64. d	65. c	66. c
67. d	68. c	69. c	70. c	71. b	72. a
73. b	74. c	75. c	76. d	77. c	78. b
79. c	80. d	81. d	82. a	83. b	84. d
85. c	86. a	87. c	88. d	89. b	90. c
91. c					

Answers   167

3 Peripheral neurophysiology

1. c	2. c	3. c	4. c	5. c	6. d
7. a	8. c	9. a	10. d	11. c	12. b
13. b	14. a	15. b	16. b	17. d	18. d
19. c	20. c	21. b	22. c	23. b	24. b
25. c	26. a	27. c	28. a	29. a	30. d
31. b	32. c	33. a	34. d	35. a	36. a
37. c	38. b	39. c	40. d	41. c	

4 Central neurophysiology

1. a	2. d	3. d	4. c	5. a	6. d
7. c	8. b	9. c	10. a	11. c	12. d
13. d	14. d	15. b	16. c	17. a	18. d
19. a	20. a	21. c	22. a	23. b	24. b
25. a	26. d	27. b	28. c	29. b	30. d
31. b	32. a	33. d	34. b	35. b	36. b
37. b	38. d	39. c	40. b	41. d	42. d
43. b	44. a	45. b			

5 Sensory physiology

1. b	2. b	3. c	4. c	5. b	6. a
7. c	8. d	9. b	10. b	11. c	12. d
13. d	14. d	15. a	16. c	17. c	18. d
19. a	20. a	21. c	22. a	23. d	24. d
25. d	26. c	27. b	28. a	29. b	30. d
31. d	32. b	33. d	34. b	35. b	36. b
37. c	38. b	39. d	40. b	41. c	42. c
43. c	44. c	45. d	46. b	47. c	48. c
49. c	50. b	51. a	52. a	53. b	54. d
55. c	56. b	57. b	58. d	59. c	60. d
61. b	62. a	63. c	64. d	65. d	

6 Autonomic nervous system

1. d	2. c	3. b	4. b	5. b	6. b
7. a	8. c	9. a	10. d	11. a	12. c
13. c	14. d	15. a	16. c	17. a	18. d
19. d	20. c	21. d	22. b	23. c	24. c

25. a	26. d	27. d	28. c	29. d	30. d
31. a	32. d	33. b	34. a	35. a	36. b
37. a	38. c	39. c	40. a	41. b	42. d
43. c	44. d	45. d	46. b	47. d	48. d
49. c	50. d	51. d	52. d	53. b	54. a
55. d	56. d	57. c	58. c	59. a	60. c
61. c	62. b	63. a	64. c	65. c	66. c
67. a	68. a	69. b	70. b	71. b	72. d
73. b	74. d	75. a	76. c	77. a	78. a
79. c	80. b	81. a			

7 Gastrointestinal physiology

1. b	2. a	3. d	4. c	5. c	6. d
7. c	8. d	9. c	10. d	11. a	12. a
13. d	14. b	15. a	16. c	17. d	18. b
19. b	20. c	21. b	22. d	23. b	24. d
25. b	26. c	27. a	28. c	29. a	30. c
31. d	32. d	33. c	34. b	35. d	36. c
37. d	38. d	39. c	40. a	41. b	42. a
43. a	44. a	45. c	46. b	47. a	48. a
49. a	50. c	51. c	52. c	53. d	54. b
55. a	56. d	57. a	58. c	59. d	60. b
61. a	62. a	63. c	64. d	65. c	66. b
67. c	68. d	69. a	70. a	71. a	

8 Cardiovascular physiology

1. d	2. d	3. a	4. a	5. a	6. b
7. c	8. b	9. d	10. d	11. d	12. b
13. b	14. c	15. a	16. d	17. c	18. b
19. a	20. d	21. a	22. c	23. c	24. a
25. b	26. c	27. c	28. d	29. c	30. a
31. c	32. a	33. a	34. a	35. c	36. c
37. d	38. c	39. b	40. d	41. c	42. c
43. c	44. d	45. c	46. d	47. d	48. b
49. d	50. d	51. b	52. c	53. d	54. a
55. c	56. c	57. c	58. b	59. d	60. b
61. b	62. a	63. c	64. c	65. c	66. b
67. c	68. c	69. b	70. a	71. a	72. c
73. c	74. b	75. c	76. a	77. c	78. a

Answers   169

79. d	80. b	81. d	82. b	83. a	84. d
85. d	86. c	87. a	88. b	89. b	90. a
91. d	92. d	93. a	94. b	95. c	96. a
97. d	98. a	99. b	100. a	101. d	102. b
103. c	104. c	105. d	106. d	107. c	108. c
109. b	110. b	111. c	112. a	113. a	114. d
115. c					

9 Respiratory physiology

1. c	2. c	3. a	4. b	5. b	6. c
7. c	8. d	9. d	10. d	11. d	12. d
13. c	14. a	15. c	16. c	17. d	18. b
19. b	20. c	21. b	22. a	23. b	24. c
25. a	26. c	27. d	28. a	29. b	30. a
31. d	32. d	33. d	34. b	35. d	36. d
37. b	38. d	39. b	40. d	41. d	42. a
43. b	44. a	45. c	46. a	47. c	48. c
49. b	50. d	51. b	52. a	53. b	54. c
55. d	56. b	57. a	58. a	59. b	60. b
61. c	62. c	63. b	64. c	65. c	66. d
67. a	68. b	69. c	70. d	71. c	72. c
73. c	74. b	75. b	76. b	77. b	78. d
79. b	80. b	81. a	82. a	83. d	84. a
85. a	86. b	87. a	88. a	89. d	90. b
91. a					

10 Renal physiology

1. b	2. c	3. c	4. c	5. c	6. a
7. a	8. c	9 c	10. b	11. c	12. b
13. c	14. a	15. c	16. b	17. a	18. c
19. a	20. a	21. d	22. a	23. c	24. b
25. c	26. c	27. b	28. b	29 d	30. d
31. a	32. c	33. a	34. c	35. c	36. a
37. d	38. d	39 a	40. b	41. d	42. b
43. b	44. a	45. a	46. d	47. b	48. d
49. c	50. a	51. c	52. c	53. d	54. d
55. d	56. d	57. d	58. c	59. c	60. a
61. c	62. a				

11 Endocrinology

1. b	2. d	3. b	4. a	5. a	6. b
7. b	8. c	9. b	10. a	11. a	12. b
13. c	14. b	15. a	16. a	17. a	18. a
19. b	20. b	21. a	22. c	23. a	24. b
25. a	26. d	27. a	28. d	29. c	30. b
31. b	32. b	33. b	34. d	35. d	36. c
37. b	38. a	39. b	40. d	41. d	42. d
43. d	44. a	45. b	46. a	47. c	48. c
49. b	50. c	51. b	52. c	53. d	54. b
55. c	56. c	57. a	58. d	59. a	60. c
61. c	62. a	63. c	64. c	65. c	66. b
67. b	68. a	69. b	70. d	71. b	72. a
73. d	74. a	75. d	76. a	77. d	78. b
79. a	80. a	81. c	82. b	83. b	84. d
85. a	86. a	87. d	88. c	89. b	90. d
91. d	92. c	93. a			

12 Reproductive physiology

1. d	2. a	3. d	4. a	5. d	6. c
7. c	8. a	9. c	10. d	11. b	12. a
13. d	14. c	15. d	16. b	17. c	18. d
19. c	20. a	21. c	22. a	23. d	24. a
25. b	26. d	27. c	28. c	29. c	30. b
31. c	32. d	33. c	34. c	35. b	36. b
37. a	38. a	39. c	40. a	41. d	42. b
43. b	44. d	45. c	46. b	47. b	48. c
49. a	50. c	51. b	52. c	53. b	54. b
55. d	56. c	57. c	58. b	59. b	60. d
61. c	62. d				